Yoruba Traditional Practices
versus
Orthodox Western Medicine

Dr. Olayioye Oluwole Odetayo
B.Sc., M.B., Ch.B., FMCS, FWACS.

Copyright © 2022 Olayioye Oluwole Odetayo

This publication may not be reproduced, stored in a retrieval system, or transmitted in whole or part, in any form or by any means, electronic, mechanical, photocopying, recording or otherwise without prior written permission of the publisher. All rights reserved solely by the author/publisher.

Yoruba Traditional Practices versus Orthodox Western Medicine Written by Dr. Olayioye Oluwole Odetayo

Illustrations and cover design by Oluwaseyi A. Alade. ©

All rights reserved.

ISBN: 9798369661338

Publisher:
Adetola Specialist Clinics Ltd
9 Williams street, Ifako, Gbagada,
P.O. Box 475, Shomolu, Lagos.
+234-7080866144
+234-8030898105

All rights reserved.

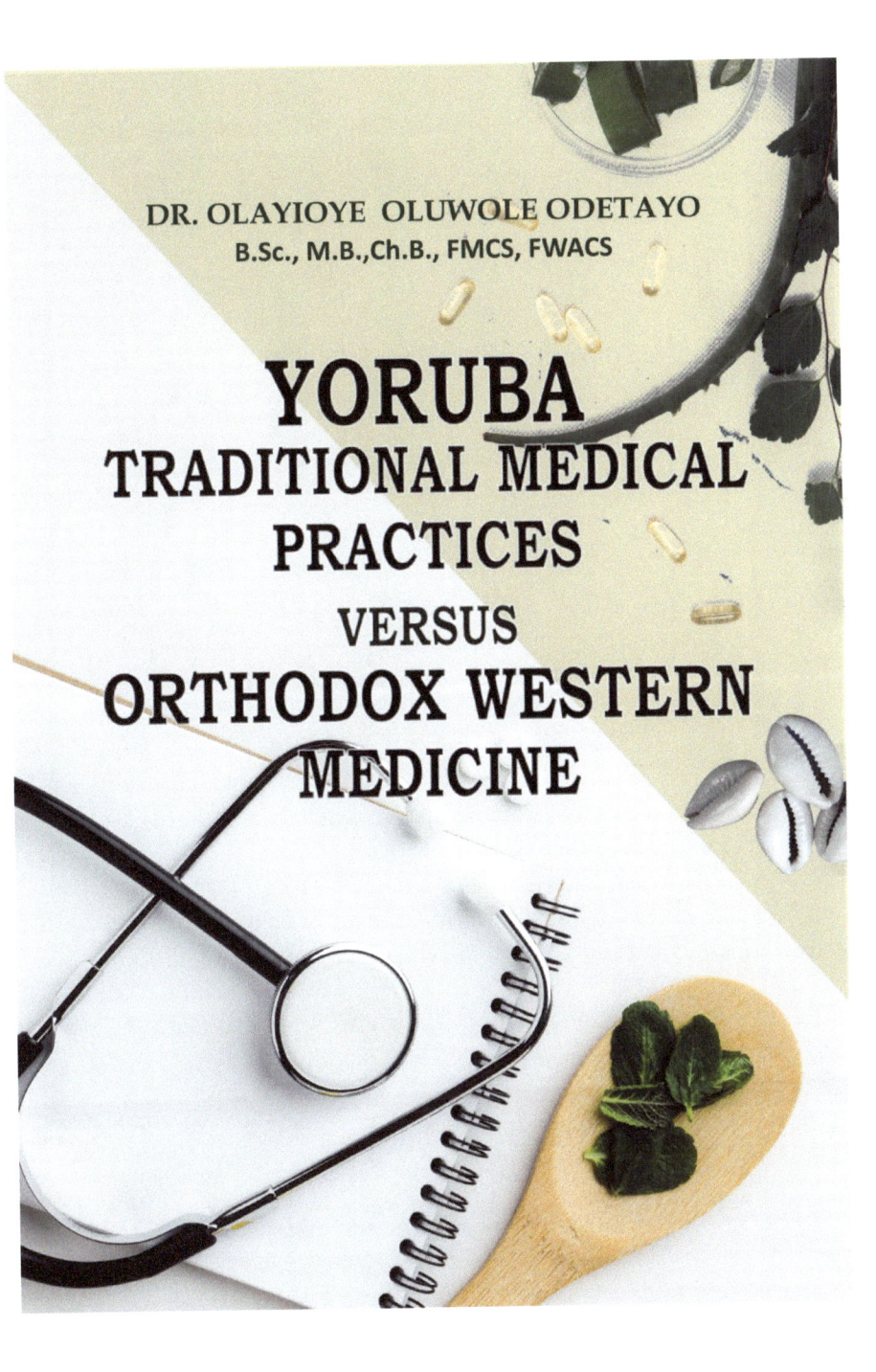

Dr. Olayioye Oluwole Odetayo

ACKNOWLEDGMENTS

My gratitude goes to the following people who offered useful suggestions in the writing of this book:

Late Pa Abraham Ojo (Ojus Photos of Gbongan), an uncle of mine, who answered some questions on traditional practices before his death.

Mrs Enitan Odetayo Tanimowo, my daughter, for her useful suggestions.

Pa. V. Olufemi Adefela, founding editor-in-chief of News Agency of Nigeria and Pan-African News Agency.

Artist Oluwaseyi A. Alade, who illustrated the diagrams in this book.

My special gratitude to ALMIGHTY GOD for the gift of life. He made everything possible.

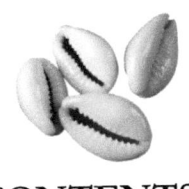

CONTENTS

	Introduction	i
1	Antenatal care	1
2	Child delivery and postnatal care	7
3	Circumcision	13
4	Child nutrition	17
5	Family planning	21
6	Polygamy	25
7	Superstitions	29
8	Traditional bone treatment	33
9	Traditional & Orthodox Mental care	39
10	Faith healing	47
11	*Abiku*	55
12	Appendix- Tribal marks in Yorubaland	63

Dr. Olayioye Oluwole Odetayo

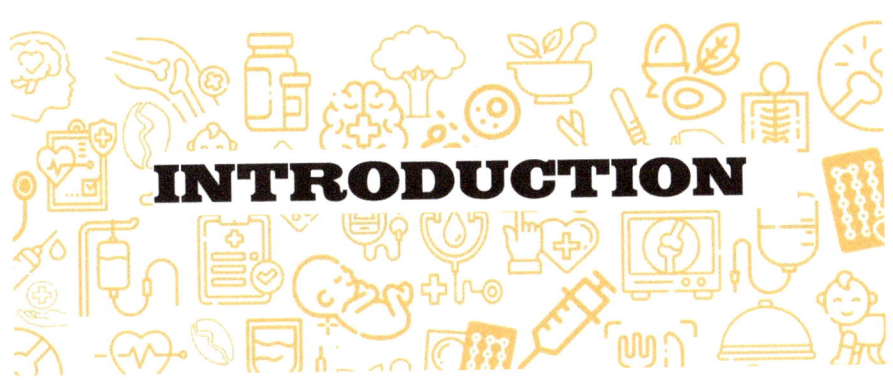

INTRODUCTION

I qualified as a Medical Practitioner in 1979 and have practiced up to date mostly in South-West Nigeria among the Yoruba people of west Africa. I was born and bred in this region and so I understand many of the traditional practices of my people.

In the 1950s and 1960s when I was growing up, there were a few government hospitals in the big cities in South-West Nigeria. These hospitals named General Hospitals were located in cities such as Lagos, Ibadan, Ile-Ife, Ilesha etc. The smaller towns like Gbongan, where I was born, had maternity centres and dispensaries manned by midwives and dispensary assistants.

These health institutions were supplemented by mission hospitals such as the Seventh Day Adventist Hospital, Ile-Ife, Wesley Guild Hospital, Ilesha and ECWA Hospital in Egbe in present day Kogi State. University College Hospital, Ibadan was already in existence by then. I can remember my father accompanying his aunt, Mama Alice, to UCH in early 1960s for some serious ailment. Very serious cases, especially when surgeries were necessary, were taken to these big hospitals.

Due to the poor economic status of most families, few individuals could afford medical treatment in these health institutions. Many ailments were treated in-house by families with herbal concoctions (called *Agbo*).

Only serious sicknesses were taken to these various health institutions. I remember having acute malaria in 1965 and was treated with concoctions for a couple of weeks in the village. This necessitated my missing classes in school then.

Most child deliveries were taken by experienced grandmothers in-house with sometimes disastrous outcomes. But difficult labour cases would be taken to these hospitals if the families could raise funds to cover medical treatment. My father told me in his old age how my mother had prolonged labour and had to be taken to the Seventh Day Hospital, Ile-Ife, where I was born in 1952.

Based upon my understanding of many traditional medical practices, I have been able to compare these practices with orthodox western medicine. Many of these practices are discussed in the various chapters.

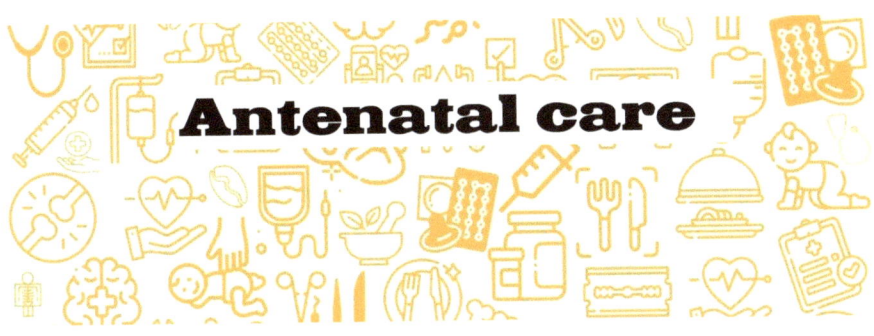

Antenatal care

1

Antenatal care, that is medical care for pregnant women, was barely available in the olden days. I guess that herbal concoctions were given to pregnant women by families. The delivery was taken by grandmothers, who were quite experienced. Babies were cleaned with various local concoctions or creams applied to the body. The baby's head would be moulded by hand, and this could have caused brain damage to the newborn. The newborn was force-fed with herbal concoctions (*Agbo*) soon after birth, which could cause aspiration pneumonia. The umbilical cord was cut with crude instruments. I can remember my father preparing sharp instruments from palm fronds. Dressing of the umbilicus was done with blackish creams and mentholated balm, when available. The newborn was thus exposed to infection of the umbilicus or even general septicaemia. With inadequate medical care, such infection was a death sentence to the newborn.

Antenatal care and Infant & Child Welfare were the main components of Primary Health Care in Nigeria since the early 1970s. In 1976, I started my student Clinical Postings in the Primary Health Centres in Ile-Ife. The first injection I gave was at the Child Welfare Clinic at Ilare Maternity Home, Ile-Ife, under the supervision of the late Professor Adeniyi-Jones, a renowned Community Health

Physician.

Despite the fall in the quality of health care in Nigeria over the past fifty years, subsequent governments have maintained good antenatal care and child welfare at the Primary Health Centres. Vaccines are given at these health centres free of charge. The health care of children have therefore improved over the years.

The good outcome of immunization of pregnant women and infants has been the disappearance of various childhood diseases. Tetanus infection in newborns, older children and adults has become a rarity in the big cities since the 1990s. Yearly measles outbreak among children has also become rare.

For mothers, good pregnancy outcome has been the norm now with the availability of modern medical care. Stillbirths have become rare with the availability of government and private hospitals. Also, maternal mortality and morbidity have reduced considerably with the wide availability of secondary and tertiary hospitals that offer good medical services. In the olden days, such medical centres were only available in a few big cities.

Traditional Birth Attendants (TBAs) came into prominence in the 1980s especially in the rural areas and smaller towns. Their presence is also noticed in low socio-economic areas of the big towns and cities. TBAs are usually poorly educated elderly women who are experienced in the care of pregnant women and child delivery. Most of them have undergone trainings by WHO and other health Agencies from the various certificates they hang in their practices. These trainings are usually of short durations, i.e. days and weeks. They give pregnant women various concoctions (sometimes called '**Aseje**'). These concoctions are said to make the babies strong and prepare the women for safe delivery. A few of these TBAs in the cities have worked in hospitals as low level staffs and they sometimes give tablets and injections, particularly Tetanus vaccine. They are said to be close to communities and trusted by them. Their charges for antenatal care and child deliveries are quite cheap when compared with what obtains in hospitals and Health centres manned by skilled health workers. They are to refer difficult cases to Hospitals for prompt care by skilled health workers. However, our experience is they usually delay difficult cases before referral and this could have disastrous consequences on babies and their mothers. Many TBAs complain of difficulty in collecting money from referred patients and discrimination against them by trained midwives and doctors because of their low educational levels. In the 1980s and early 1990s, many of the referred women in labour from TBAs had raw leaves inserted into their birth canals. However, this practice has simply disappeared. This must be due to the various trainings from international and government agencies. Thus infections of new born babies and mothers have automatically reduced. Many churches have also set up maternity centres usually run by Traditional Birth Attendants.

Christian missionaries introduced modern orthodox medical care in many parts of Nigeria. The Seventh Day Adventists (SDA) established a Hospital at Ile-Ife, Osun State, in 1940. Coincidentally, I had the good fortune of being born in this hospital in 1952. My father, in his old age, told me the circumstances of my birth. He said that my mother had been in prolonged labour before she was taken to the SDA hospital where I was delivered. Without such an action, I could have been part of the statistics of stillbirths and my mother could have died during her first pregnancy.

Unfortunately, the Yorubas believed such a woman was an *Emere*, meaning someone with a familiar spirit who had probably promised her coven to die with her first pregnancy. There is so much stupidity in some of our cultural beliefs! Apart from being born at the Seventh Day Adventist Hospital, Ile-Ife, I can remember having an incision of a large abscess on my right ankle in 1959 at the hospital. A white doctor operated on me using a brilliant lamp for the procedure. I remember wondering why I had no pain during the procedure and concluded that it was the brilliant light he used to remove the pain of an otherwise painful procedure.

The Wesley Guild Hospital, Ilesha, Osun State, was built by the Methodist Church in the early part of the 20th century. The hospital was later taken over by the University of Ife Teaching Hospitals Complex in the 1970s when I had some clinical postings at this hospital both as a clinical student and as an intern. Even before the takeover by the Teaching Hospital, the hospital was well known internationally for paediatric and medical care and research. Some of the medical research conducted was on *"Ijesha Shake"* by the renowned neurologist, late Professor B. O. Oshuntokun. *Ijesha Shake* was a neurological illness that presented itself yearly with convulsions and coma. Initially, the disease was thought to be a viral illness because of its seasonal occurrence. But a colleague and friend, Dr Bola Adamolekun, proved that the presentation of the disease was similar to vitamin B6 [Pyridoxine] deficiency. He proved that the seasonal outbreak was because the people with low levels of the vitamin ate *Ekuku*, a butterfly larva, that was available during the rainy season. An enzyme in the insect consumed the little available vitamin in the body, thus producing avitaminosis with its clinical presentation of convulsions and coma.

Another popular Missionary Hospital during my growing up years was ECWA Hospital, Egbe, in present-day Kogi state, Nigeria. Many of the missionary doctors in these hospitals were specialists who could carry out many medical and surgical procedures.

Yoruba Traditional Practices versus Orthodox Western Medicine

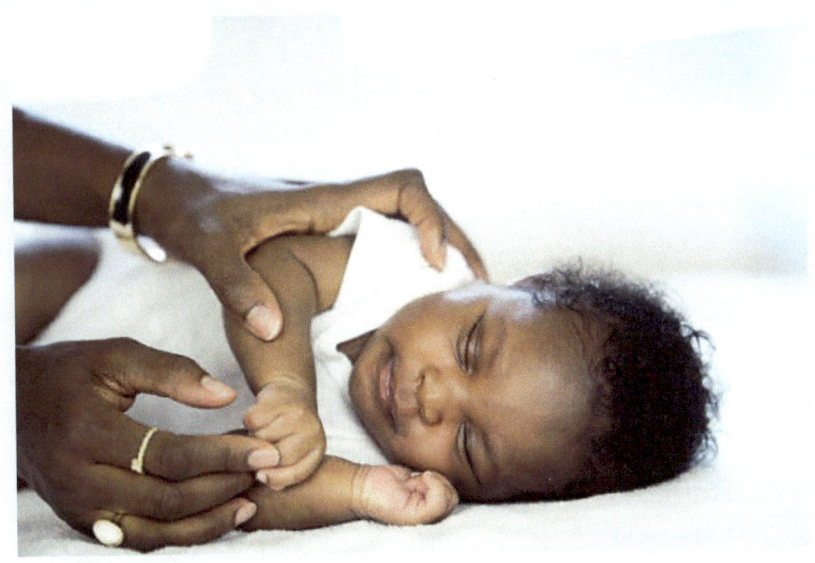

References.

1. Adamolekun B. (1992). A seasonal ataxic syndrome in South-Western Nigeria: An etiological hypothesis of acute thiamine defiency. Ethnic. Dis. 2(2):185-186.

2. Ashiru M. O. (1988). The food value of larvae of Anaphe venata Bulter (Lepidoptera: Notodontidae). Ecology of Food and Nutrition, 22:313-320.

3. Oshuntokun B. O. (1972). Epidemic Ataxia in Western Nigeria. BMJ 2:589.

4. Pearson C. A., Moore D. L. and David-West T. S. (1973). Virus studies in "Ilesha Shakes". W. Afr. Med. J. 22(1):20-22.

5. Bolanle Adamolekun, David W. Macandless & Roger F. Butterworth. (1997) Metabolic Brain Disease 12, 251-258.

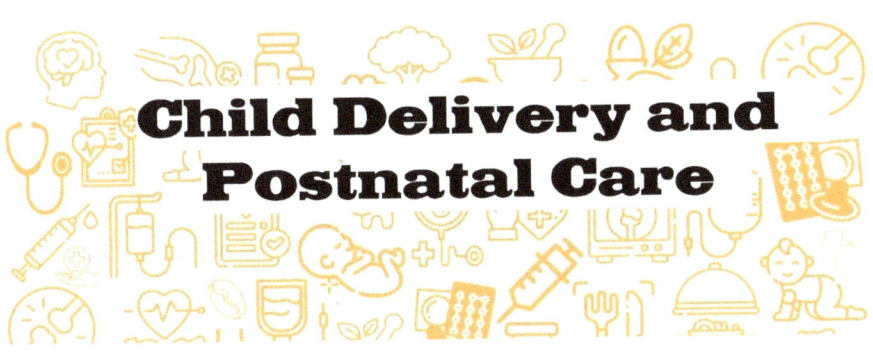

Child Delivery and Postnatal Care

2

Traditional practices.

Stillbirths were common in the olden days when surgical delivery was non-existent. There must have been high maternal mortality and morbidity also. I am sure the traditional spiritualists/herbalists (**Babalawos**) would have been involved in many difficult deliveries. I am not sure that incantations or concoctions can widen a narrow pelvis or birth canal for a big baby. I read in an article years ago of spiritualists in East Africa who performed caesarian sections on women with obstructed labour. To control the bleeding as in normal operations on the uterus, the surgeon would be chewing special leaves which would be spewed on the wound. Even if the babies came out alive, few women would have survived the surgery. Thank God for orthodox western medicine, child delivery has become easier with good outcomes for both the baby and the mother.

Each family in *Yorubaland* had the standard care for pregnant women:

- I remember that in my childhood days, a special soup was given to women who just gave birth to babies. The soup was called

'Ate' (meaning tasteless) and was prepared with melon seed, bitter leaf, smoked fish, locust beans and hot spices. It had no salt or red palm oil added. I enjoyed eating this soup because the fish made it tasty. Scientifically, the low salt in the soup is good for the post-partum period to help the women eliminate the excess fluid accumulated in the body during pregnancy. The hot pepper is a helpful analgesic for a woman who just delivered. With the early death of my mother, this practice was not continued in my generation.

- A common practice I disagree with is the use of hot water to press the lower abdomen of women who just delivered. My dad's aunt, Mama Alice, was very good at using very hot water to press any sore area of the body. Some women would have suffered some degrees of skin burns. Many women would have had postpartum haemorrhage and I am sure there would have been various concoctions to take care of this. But many women would have died.

- In my early years, my father used to mention a special disease of women called *'Igbalode'*, that killed fast. I believe that this disease is Menorrhagia/Metrorrhagia which involves heavy bleeding from a woman's womb, sometimes without an obvious cause. Many women would have died from severe blood loss. Special concoctions would be given to affected women. Miscarriages of pregnancies would have been common, too, with its sequella of heavy blood loss and sometimes death of the woman.

The care of the newborn baby was not too good with certain bad practices such as:

- The cutting of the umbilical cord was unhygienic. The care of the umbilical stump was done badly with the application of unhygienic black paste. *Ori* (shea butter cream) and mentholated balm were also applied. These are all good sources of local sepsis or even generalized infection. They contributed to the high infant mortality rate that was in existence before the advent of orthodox western medicine.

- The inside of houses were beautified with mixtures of ground leaves, charcoal and goat faeces. Animal faeces are known to habour Tetanus spores which can easily contaminate wounds in both children and adults.

- At naming or christening celebrations, everybody would want to carry the baby who was regarded as a bundle of joy. This is discouraged in orthodox medical practice to prevent the newborn from getting infected.

- Yoruba women carry newborn babies on the back soon after delivery. This act provides good warmth for the newborn. In my medical practice, we have advised mothers who could not afford to seek incubator care for their premature babies to use this method and many of the babies have survived. Using the Kangaroo bag to carry babies is an alternative in modern times.

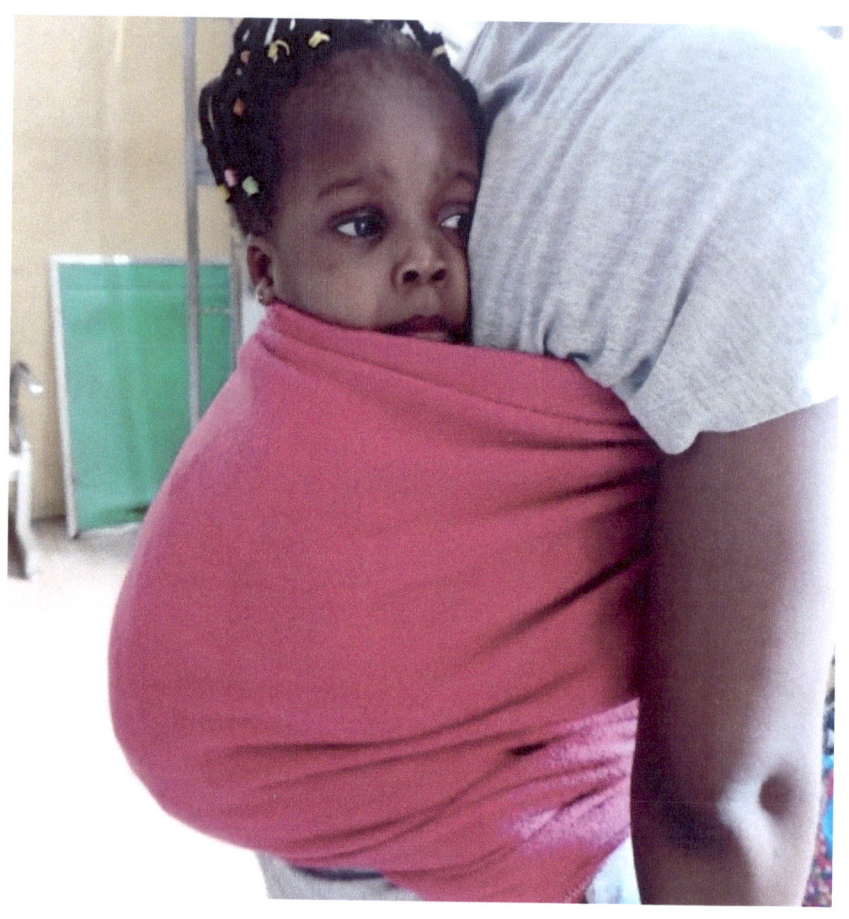

A baby being carried on the back of her mother.

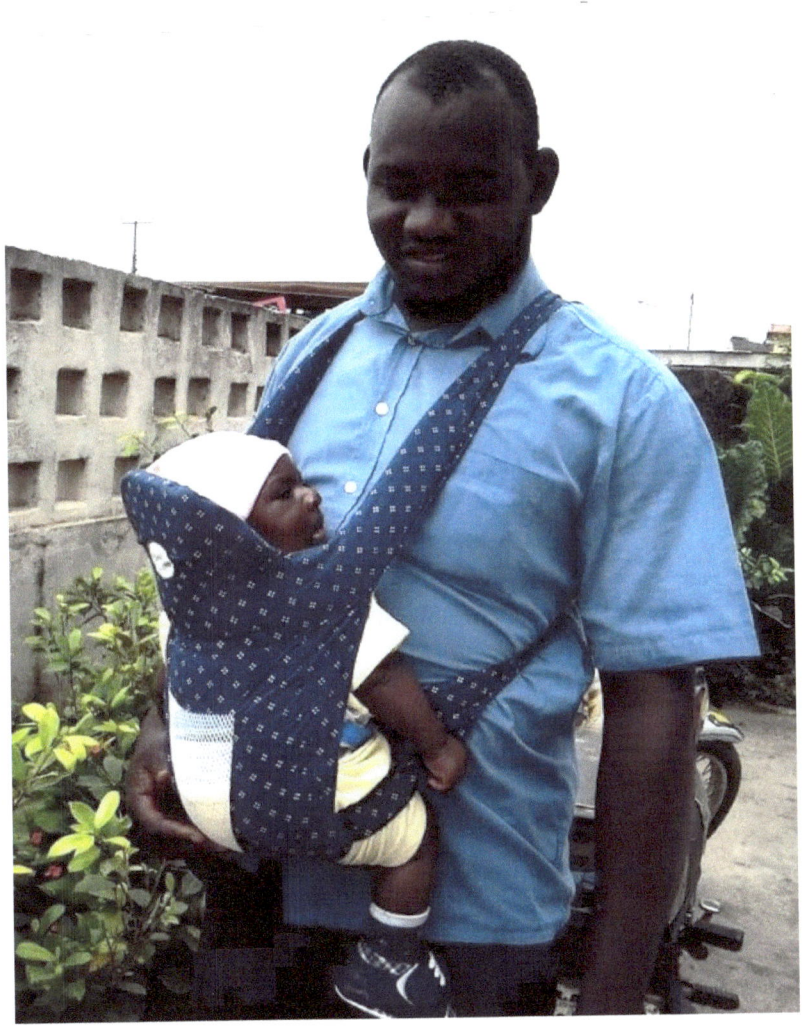

A baby being carried with a Kangaroo bag.

References.

1. Odetayo Olayioye Oluwole (2020) MY ODYSSEY – Autobiography Of An African Surgeon
2. World Health Organization. (2000) "General guidelines for methodologies on research and evaluation of traditional medicine."
3. United Nations Population Fund (1996): Evaluation, Findings: Support to traditional birth attendants. http://www.unfpa.org/pdfn-issue7.pdf
4. World Vision: Ethiopia: Trained traditional birth attendants easing delivery. (2011)
5. Ray, AM; Salihu HM (2004). "The impact of maternal mortality interventions using traditional birth attendants and village midwives." J. Obstet Gynaecol 24(1):5-11
6. Iyaniwura CA, Yussuf Q. Utilization of antenatal care and delivery services in Sagamu, south western Nigeria. African Journal of Reproductive Health. 2009; 13(2):111-122.
7. Doctor HV. Intergenerational differences in antenatal care and supervised deliveries in Nigeria. Health and Place. 2011; 17: 480-489s.

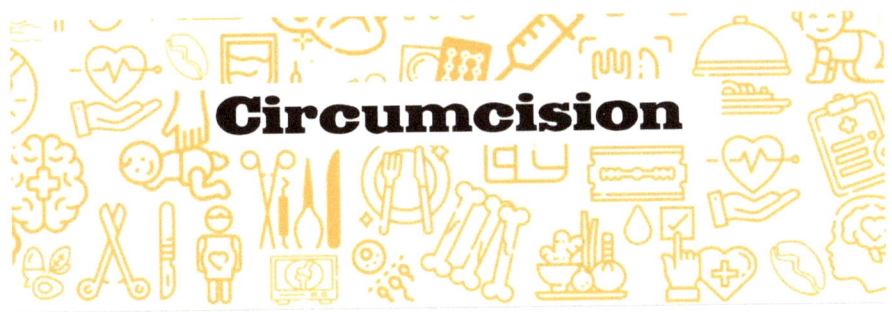

Circumcision

3

Circumcision is the surgical removal of the skin covering the tip of the penis. In Yoruba culture, child circumcision is usually done for male children soon after birth. There are specialists in performing circumcision on children called *'akomonila'*. The same people make tribal marks on children. In my growing-up years, I watched many cases of circumcision done on male children.

The *akomonila* comes with his crude instruments wrapped in a dirty cloth. These instruments are made by the local blacksmith and are not sterile. The whole procedure is also unsterile. The *akomonila* washes his hands and the instruments used with ordinary water at the end of the procedure and leaves. A local black cream would be applied to the wound thereafter. I am not sure there was an answer to occasional cases of heavy bleeding from circumcision as it happens in children with bleeding disorders.

Some other cultures carry out circumcision on grown-up children or even adults. I learnt that in some African cultures, circumcision of the males is a rite of passage into adulthood. In the Midwest States of Nigeria, I understand that circumcision of the female child is part of the marriage rite.

Orthodox western medicine recommends circumcision for the male child for hygienic purposes. Incidences of penile cancers are said to be reduced in circumcised males. Incidence of HIV spread is also said to be reduced in circumcised males. The standard medical practice is to carry out the surgery on a neonate with or without anaesthesia. In recent years, the use of plastic rings, called **Plastibel**, is common in hospitals. It is particularly useful in children under one year of life. It reduces bleeding in all cases of circumcision.

Circumcision of females is usually done by elderly women among the Yoruba people. With increasing education in the society, grandmothers are known to use tricks to circumcise young girls even when their parents are not in support. However, orthodox medicine frowns at female circumcision in babies or adults. International agencies and Human Rights groups refer to female circumcision as **Female Genital Mutilation** to show disdain for the procedure. Many governments all over the world, including Africa, have outlawed this practice.

Many women circumcised as babies have presented as adults in hospitals with complications from badly done procedures. The common one is extensive scarring of the vulva and labia. My understanding of female circumcision is cutting the tip or even the body of the clitoris. Many of the procedures done by traditional practitioners or grandmothers go beyond the cutting of the clitoris to involve cutting the minor and major labia.

The result of extensive scarring of the perineum is difficulty in child delivery. Many women also report reduced sexual enjoyment with the cutting of the clitoris. Many of the babies circumscribed using unhygienic instruments would have been infected and possibly died from infections such as tetanus.

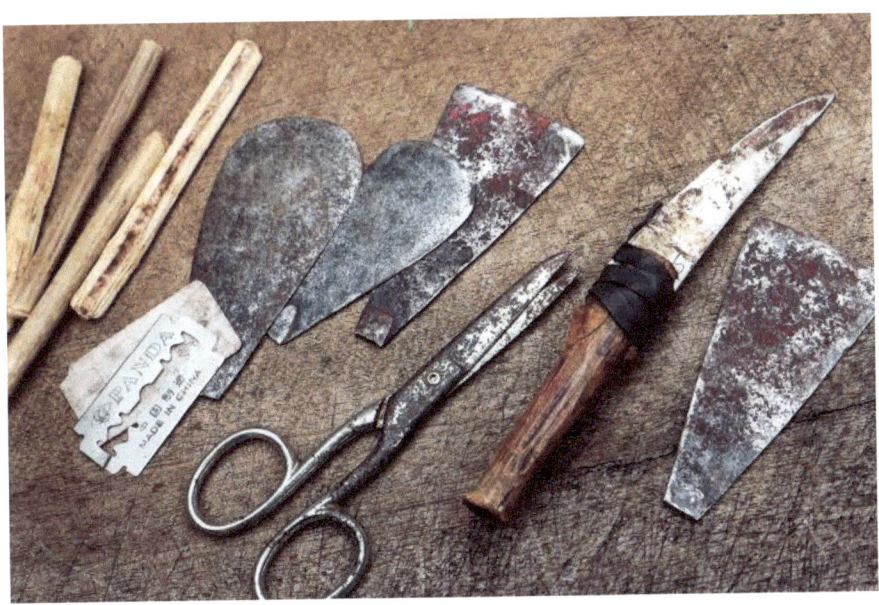

Crude traditional tools used for Female GenitalCircumcision.

References.

1. Female Genital Mutilation/Cutting: A Global Concern UNICEF, New York, 2016.

2. Female Genital Mutilation. Who.int

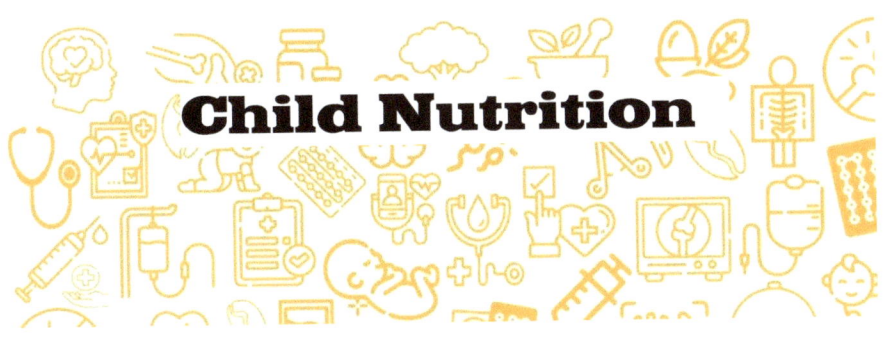

Child Nutrition

4

Like all mammalians, humans give birth to their very young babies and breastfeed them right from birth. Human breast milk is a complete meal for a newborn baby. It has enough water, nutrients and vitamins required by the baby. Hence the baby-friendly initiative of UNESCO encourages exclusive breastfeeding for a baby for the first six months of life before the introduction of cereals. African cultures encourage breastfeeding babies for up to 2 or even 3 years. There is therefore good bonding between babies and their mothers. Apart from meeting the dietary requirement of the newborn baby, protective serum passes from the mother to the baby. The baby can withstand infections better. As the baby grows, adult food is gradually introduced to the infant's diet. Some babies even demand the food they see their parents eat. At age of 1 year, most children can eat and digest adult diet.

Interestingly, in modern times, in spite of good education in the society, some women either do not breastfeed their children long enough or some even do not breastfeed their newborn babies at all. The usual reason for these women is to preserve the rounded shape of the breasts. Orthodox medicine had to step in to educate the women on the importance of breastfeeding not to the babies alone but also to the mothers. Mothers who breastfeed their babies have a good bonding with their children. In addition, breastfeeding helps to prevent the development of breast cancers in women. To maintain the good shape of their breasts, women are encouraged to use good brassieres for support. However, HIV positive mothers are advised not to breastfeed their new born babies to prevent mother-to-child transmission of the virus.

Nutritional problems usually arise when babies are weaned off the breast in traditional cultures. As discussed earlier, most food types for children in African societies lack the protein that children need for good growth. Diets in Africa are mainly starchy foods gotten from grains such as corn and millet, and tubers such as yam, cassava and cocoyam. However, there are other types of food which provide a good diet. Plantain is a good dietary component. Various types of beans are grown in Africa. These are good sources of plant protein which are of benefit to a growing child; they are usually on the food menu.

Animal meat is rare in meals for children. In my growing-up years, we were discouraged from eating chicken eggs which are very rich in protein. Proteineous insects such as flying termites were forbidden to us in my area, but I learnt otherwise when I went to live in present-day Ondo State of Nigeria. Elderly men went to the farms at night to scoop up bagfuls of flying termites from termite hills. These insects are then roasted for consumption and sale in the open market. Butterfly larvae, *Ekuku*, and small snails were picked on the farms and roasted or fried for eating. Among the Efiks and Ibibio of South-south Nigeria, periwinkles are part of the normal diet. These are small snails that are found in flowing rivers.

Fast-growing children need a lot of protein for growth. After the weaning of children, lack of good protein in the diet especially rich animal protein manifested as malnutrition diseases. Such diseases, including *kwashiorkor* and *marasmus*, are classified as protein energy malnutrition. Malnourished children do not grow properly and are susceptible to infections from which they die easily, especially in situations in which medical facilities are either nonexistent or unaffordable for poor families. These children either have swollen extremities and cheeks or simply remain lean with poor muscle mass. Affected children usually grow up with poorly developed brains and may not succeed in school and end up as poor unskilled labour in adult life. Poor adults may not have the wherewithal to take good care of their children in future. Thus, poverty goes from generation to generation in a vicious circle.

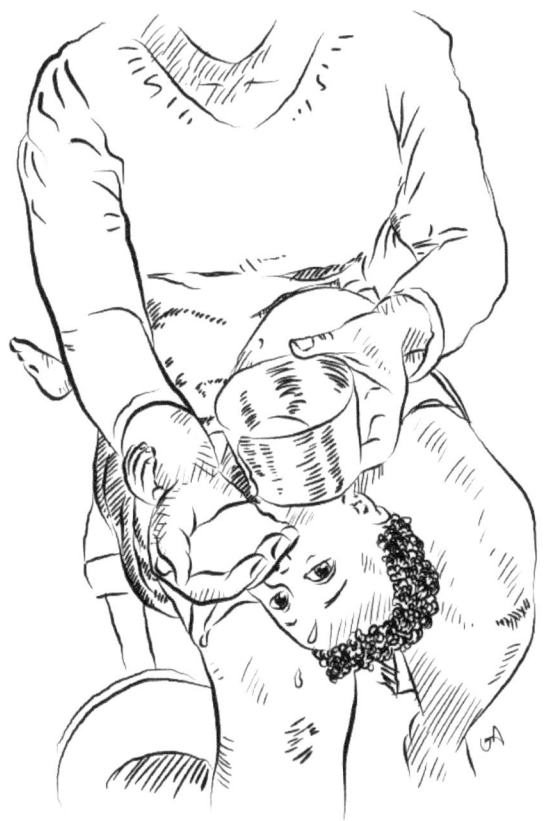

A child being force-fed.

Children being force-fed easily aspirate the food and develop pneumonia quite often. With inadequate provision of health services, many of such children have died.

References

1. Olivia Ballard and Ardythe L. Morrow. Human Milk Composition: Nutrients and bioactive Factors.. Pediatr Clin North Am. 2013 Feb. 80(1): 49-74.

2. WHO, Infant and young child nutrition. Geneva: 2003.

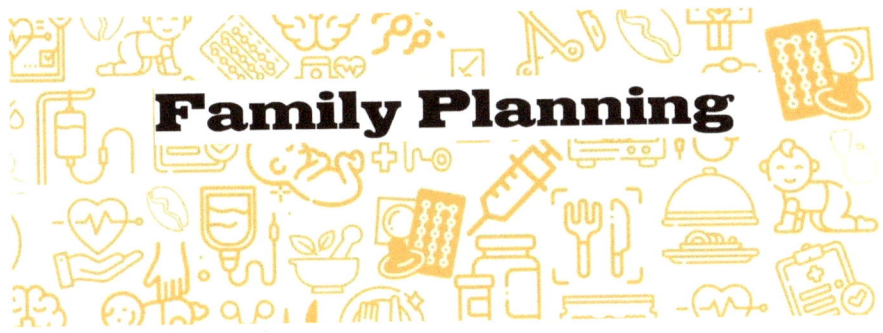

Family Planning

5

According to the World Health Organization (WHO), family planning allows individuals and couples to participate in the determining of their desired number of children and the timing of their births. It can be achieved through contraceptive methods and the treatment of involuntary infertility. The WHO is a specialized agency of the United Nations and was founded in 1947. Before the formation of the United Nations, African people had practiced family planning over the ages.

Breastfeeding is a well-known method of family planning. It suppresses ovulation in most women. Most marriages in Yorubaland were polygamous in the olden days. A man was considered to be a success when he had married many wives. High infant mortality in those days also rendered family planning unnecessary. The important thing was how many children that would survive into adulthood.

Among the moslem Hausa/Fulani of Northern Nigeria, polygamy is the norm since the Quran allows a man to marry up to four wives. I learnt during my National Youth Service year that the wives of a man in a polygamous home took turns in sharing the night with their husbands. Each wife had a day to cook for the man and share his bed at night. With little understanding of the local language, I could not find out more about child survival rates among the local people. But I observed that women breastfed their children in infancy till they could tolerate adult diet. However, the local diet appeared poor to me. The diet consisted mainly of grains - rice, maize and millet. An example of a soup I tasted was from dried Baobab tree leaves, with tiny pieces of meat and drops of groundnut oil. I am not sure if animal meat is part of their local diet as they were rural *Fulanis* who reared animals for sale. I have not interacted closely with the Ibos from Eastern Nigeria. But I have eaten their soups many times. Their soups are varied and rich, loaded with meat and dried stockfish. The major staple foods are Cassava, yam and plantain.

In *Yoruba* land, I believe there must have been herbalists (*Babalawos*) that are experts in family planning. In my early years of practice as a medical doctor, I was told about two women who were each given special family planning rings to prevent pregnancy. The ring was said to have been effective in one of them with no pregnancy over many years, but it failed in the second woman.

In modern times, more women are coming forward for family planning in clinics and hospitals. A couple of decades earlier, many men prevented their wives from going for family planning for fear that they may become promiscuous. But in recent years, most husbands encourage their wives to go for family planning or even follow them to the hospital. The men would say that they cannot afford to have too many children to care for, especially with regard to paying for their education. In the generation of my children, young couples are now having one or two kids. It is an aphorism in medical circles that the best family planning method is to educate a woman. An enlightened, educated woman will likely not have too many children. She is intelligent enough to give birth to the few children she can provide for and bring up properly.

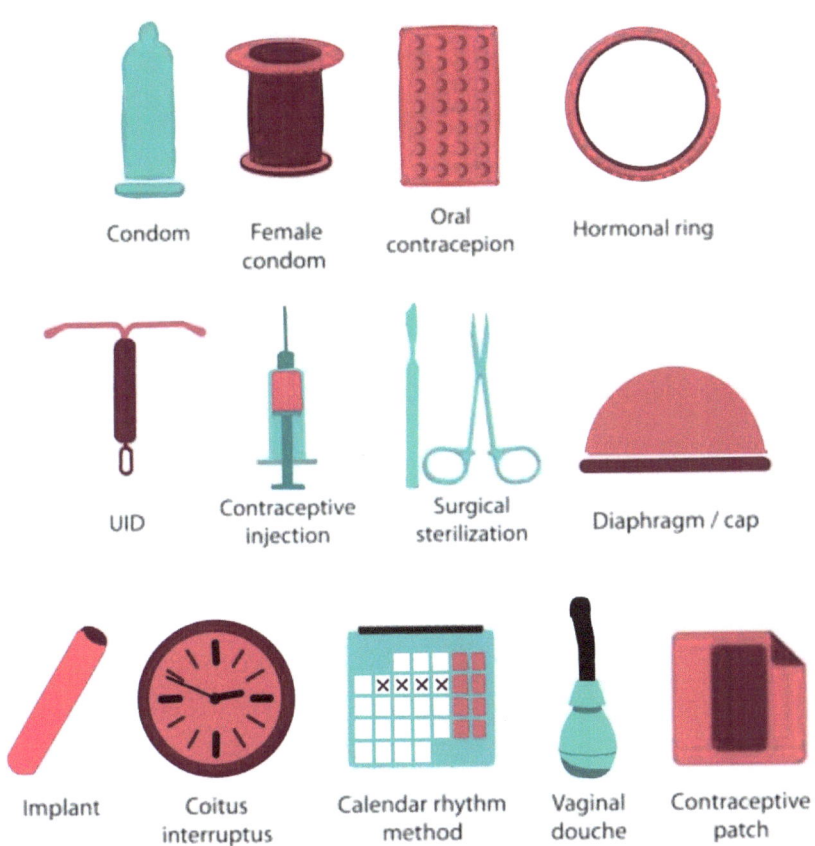

Family planning Methods

References

1. Familyplanning/contraceptionmethods. https://.who.int

2. Family Planning. https://unfpa.org.

3. Mckissack, Patricia; Mckissack, Fredrick (1995). The Royal Kingdoms of Ghana, Mali and Songhay Life in Medieval Africa. Macmillan p.104.

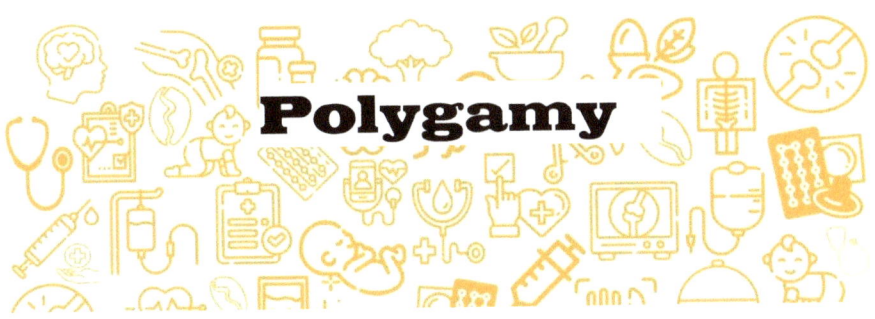

Polygamy

6

Polygamy is defined as the practice or custom of having more than one wife or husband at the same time. This was a common practice in most African tribes. There are many reasons for this in traditional societies. Some of the reasons included the following:

- Agrarian societies, as we have in South-west Nigeria, encouraged polygamy to have more people to work on the farm. Farmers usually deployed their wives and children to work on their farms, especially during the planting and harvesting periods. A rich farmer with large farms would have to pay hired helpers if he did not have a large enough family.

- High infant mortality (called locally as Abiku), encouraged polygamy as a man would want to have many wives who could produce many children. Even if many of the children died early, some would survive into adulthood and carry on the family name.

- Religion: Tribes where Islam is the predominant religion do practice polygamy. The Quran, the Holy Book of Muslims, states that a man can have up to four wives. Thus, the average *muslim* usually had many wives. This is very common in Northern Nigeria, where Islam is predominant. On the other hand, Christianity preached monogamy, the practice of having one wife/husband.

In polygamous homes, total care of each child most often was the responsibility of the mother. Many of the mothers engaged in petty trading to supplement what little the man of the house gave to each of the wives. With the advent of modern education, many fathers refused to play significant roles in sending their children to school. Thus, many children from polygamous families would drop out of school to either go into full-time farming or learn trades. Economically, most of them never fared well, which in turn affected their own children too.

Monogamy in marriages is supported by modern-day living and medical science. Physical and emotional support of the children is better in monogamous homes. Proper upbringing of a few children is possible in such marriages and well-brought-up children will most probably become successful adults in the society. Sexual health is not easily compromised in monogamous relationships as against what occurs in polygamous homes.

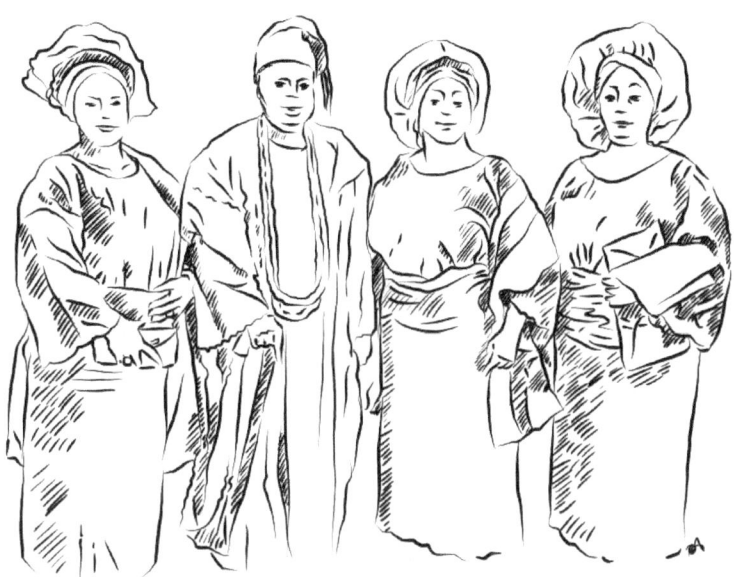

A Yoruba man and his three wives.

References

1. Kramer, Stephanie (2020). "Polygamy is rare around the world." Pew Research Centre.

2. Fenske, James. (2013) "African Polygamy, Past and Present" VoxEU.org.

3. Goody, Jack (1974) "Polygyny, Economy and the Role of Women" The Character of Kinship. Cambridge University Press. Pp. 175-190.

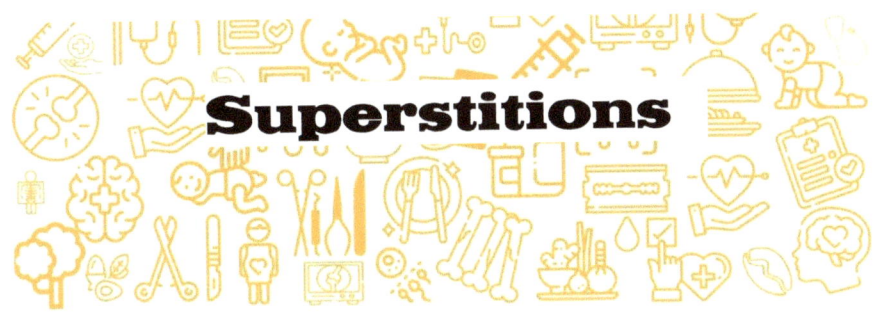

Superstitions

7

Superstitions are widely held beliefs in supernatural influences, especially, as leading to good or bad luck, or a practice based on such a belief. Superstitious beliefs are common in most African cultures. They interfere with orthodox medical management of diseases and situations a lot of time. Medical practitioners have to properly counsel affected individuals or their parents if they are minors. I shall cite a few common examples that I know and have had to counsel patients on.

1. **Moulding of a newborn's head** immediately after delivery as practiced by the Yorubas. It is believed that the head will remain flat if not moulded, thus disfiguring the growing child. In reality, the flattened head of a newborn soon becomes well rounded on its own. Medical science does not support this practice as the child can easily sustain a head injury during the moulding and this might be catastrophic.

2. **A compulsory bath of the newborn in water** is usually insisted upon. It is believed that, if this is not done, the child will have body odour throughout life. This has no scientific basis. Doctors do not encourage newborns to have early baths so as not to expose them to cold which can be injurious. Midwives usually clean bodies of newborn babies with olive oil.

3. **Forbidding children to eat eggs**. It was generally said by adults that children who ate eggs would end up as thieves in adult life. And so, we were discouraged from eating chicken eggs in our growing-up years. But we children gave ourselves nice treats whenever we picked up eggs from wandering chickens that laid eggs anywhere. Scientifically, an egg provides a balanced diet with a good source of protein that will help the child grow well. I encourage parents to give eggs to their children in their growing up years. This is very important when the children are weaned off the breast milk and are given cereals like *Akamu/Ogi* that is poor in protein. I encouraged my children to take eggs daily in their growing up years and they have fared well nutritionally.

4. **Care of the placenta after a baby is born**. The *Yorubas* regard the care of the placenta as very important and believe that it could affect a child's fortune in the future. Firstly, it is believed that a child whose placenta is eaten by a dog will end up being a thief. This has no scientific basis. I remember that my father would collect the placenta and bury it in the backyard inside a special pot. Recently, I heard that some people buy the placenta and use it for money rituals! Interestingly, Ibos do not care about the placenta after birth. I encourage parents of newborns to discard the placenta in a safe place so as not to mess up the environment.

5. **The practice of massaging any injured or painful part of the body** most often adds more injury to the situation. The commonly used shea butter (*Ori*) comes to mind. This balm is applied to any painful part of the body, usually accompanied by massaging. I advise people not to massage any injured or painful part of the body.

6. **Spirituality:** The *Yorubas* believe in rejecting negative things in their lives. While I believe in positive thinking, these people fail to accept or listen to explanations of the conditions of their

bodies. This rejection of negative things or ideas is based on their superstitious beliefs.

Even when doctors encourage people to come for medical screening, they reject such invitations. They may even add that they enjoy **divine health** and do not need to check their health status. For adequate management of many medical conditions, the doctor may need to explain to patients the possible causes and preventive methods. Many people will not listen to the explanations on how to live right so that the condition may not re-occur or how to manage the next attack better.

I grew up hearing people say *"Ori mi ko"*. (This means my head rejects it or my destiny rejects it.) With increased religiosity, the usual rhetorical response is "I reject it in Jesus name". For example, **epilepsy** is highly stigmatised and fearfully avoided among the Yoruba people. It is believed that it is contagious and runs in families. Thus, when a child is brought to the hospital while having fits, the parents usually do not accept the diagnosis and refuse any follow-up appointments after treatment.

Orthodox medicine recognizes the physical attributes of diseases and thus management is based upon the diagnosis. However, there is a strong belief in the spiritual causes of diseases among the Yoruba people. This belief system has been in the cultural systems for long and we still experience such in orthodox medical practice. Educated people usually do not exhibit this belief as much as the uneducated segments of society. However, a large segment of the population does not accept the diagnosis or the need for proper management of the condition. The effect is that many sufferers or their parents either fail to come for clinic follow-up or they seek help in the wrong places like from spiritualists.

References.

1. Ajose, Oladele A. "Preventive Medicine and Superstition in Nigeria." Africa: Journal of the International African Institute, vol. 27, no. 3 1957. Pp. 268-74 JSTOR.
2. Nasir Umar. Northeast Nigeria Myths and Superstitions Pose More Barriers to Health of Women and Babies Than Conflict. https://www.mhtf.org. 2014/06/10

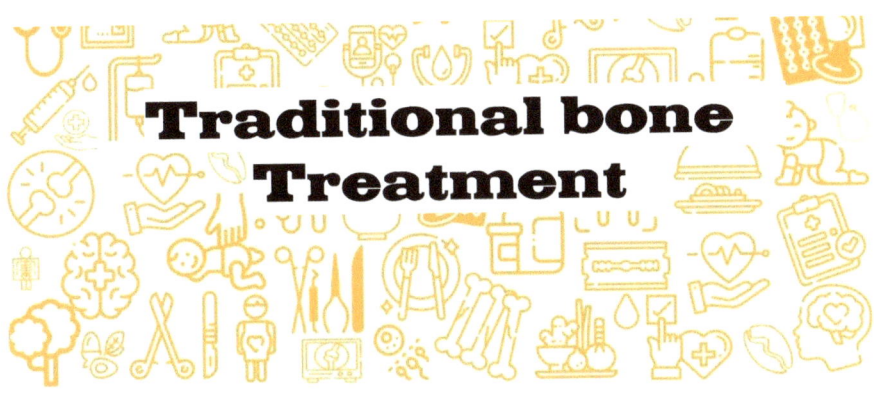

Traditional bone Treatment

8

Traditional bone setters are common in most African tribes. I have had some interactions with Yoruba and Hausa traditional bone setters. Most of the methods they use in the management of bone fractures are not scientific and they sometimes cause more injuries to the patients. Charges by traditional bone setters are far less than charges by orthodox medical practitioners thus it is quite attractive to those with poor economic means. Payments can be made in cash or even in kind.

Bone is a living tissue and will heal after injury, just like most tissues in the body. However, the duration of healing in bone is prolonged more than it is in other body tissues.

Many traditional bonesetters introduce elements of fetishism by chanting incantations while treating the broken bones. They would break chicken legs and splint them, claiming that the patients' broken bone would heal the way the chicken bone heals. These acts are done to impress the patients and their relatives. The basic requirement for healing of fractures is for the broken ends to be in contact by splinting. This splinting should be long enough for union to take place. This period could last several weeks or months depending upon the age of the patient.

Splints that are used by the traditional practitioners are usually short and most often do not immobilize the fractured part adequately. Furthermore, the splints are most often too tight, thus affecting the blood supply to the injured limbs. The resultant effect could be total loss of blood supply to the whole limb and subsequent gangrene. As an orthopaedic surgeon, I have had to amputate many limbs over the years.

In fact, many patients have died because of subsequent sepsis in some of the cases. Mal-union and non-union of fracture sites are quite common and many patients have developed short limbs. Contractures and other limb deformities also occur. Affected individuals later seek out appropriate treatment from professional orthopaedic surgeons for correction of limb deformities after wasting months and years of their lives. Sometimes the long duration from the time of the initial injury may render help too late. It is advisable that injured people with broken bones should seek help early from professional orthopaedic surgeons who have the scientific know-how and equipments for their management.

Many experts have advocated for special training for traditional bonesetters and their inclusion in the Primary Health Care system of the area or region. This will limit the many complications that do arise in the hands of traditional practitioners. I believe that this call is being hampered by the secretive nature of traditional medical practice in Africa as a whole where knowledge and expertise in the respective fields are most often passed down from generation to generation and through apprenticeships.

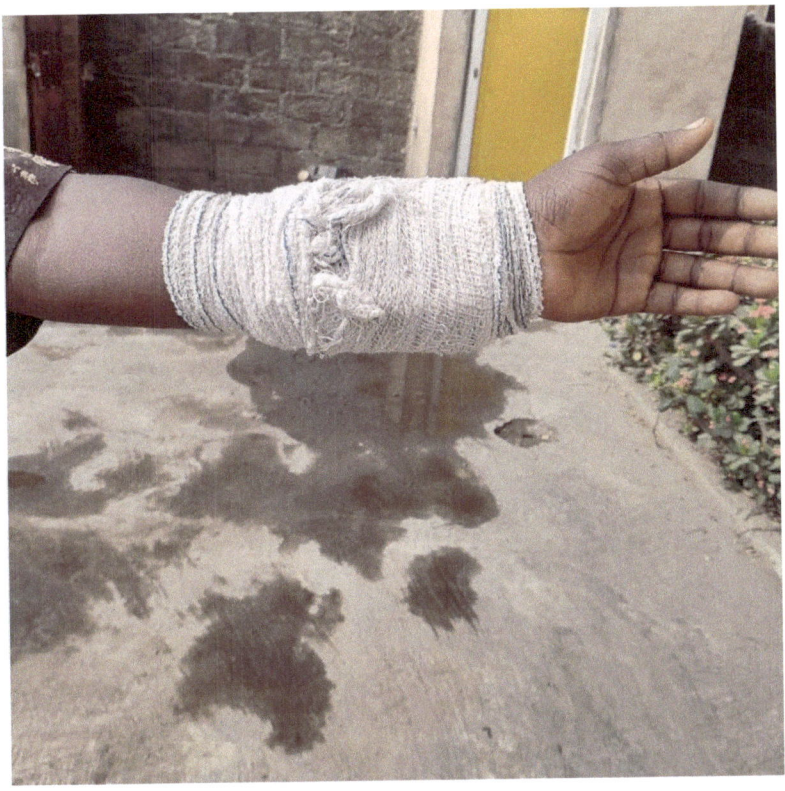

Splinting of a Forearm Fracture by A Traditional Bone Setter.

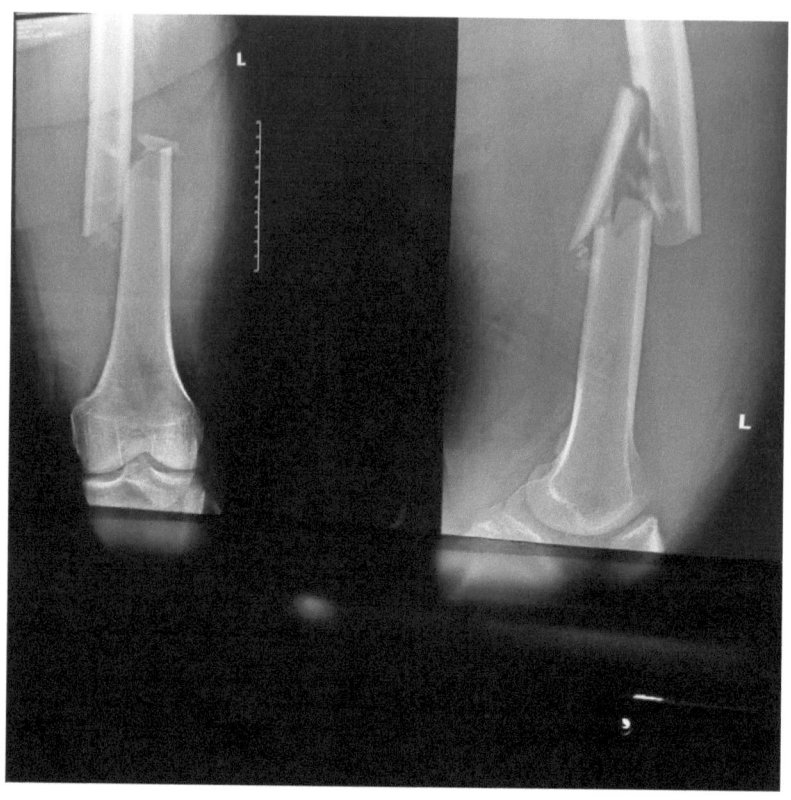

X-ray of a broken thigh bone (femur).

Yoruba Traditional Practices versus Orthodox Western Medicine

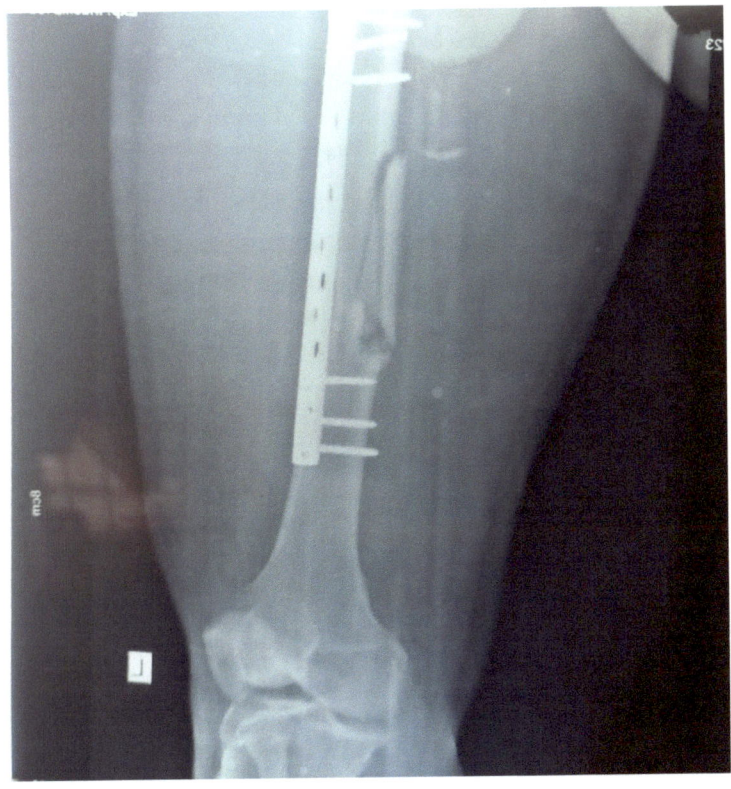

X-ray of same thigh bone after Internal Fixation with a Plate and Screws.

References.

1. A. Dada, W. Yinusa and S. O. Giwa. Review of the practice of traditional bone setting in Nigeria. Afr Health Sci. 2011 Jun; 11(2): 262-265.
2. B. Omololu, MD, S. O. Ogunlade, FRCS, and V. K. Goldasani, MBBS. The practice of Traditional Bonesetting: Training algorithin. Clin Orthop Relat Res. 2008 Oct; 466(110): 2392-2398.
3. D. A. OlaOlorun, I. O. Oladiran, A. Adeniran. Complications of fracture treatment by traditional bonesetters in southwest Nigeria. Fam Pract. 2001 Dec; 18(6): 635-7.
4. M. I. Eshete. The prevention of traditional bone setter's gangrene. The Journal of Bone and Joint Surgery. British volume 87(1), 102-103, 2005.

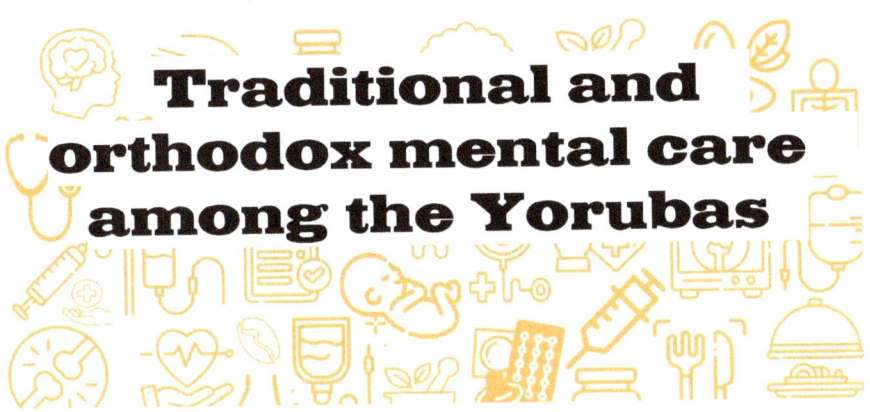

Traditional and orthodox mental care among the Yorubas

9

By **DR MOSES ABAYOMI OJO**, FMCPsych. Consultant Psychiatrist.

INTRODUCTION

Mental illnesses occur in all cultures but each culture has different perspectives regarding cause, diagnosis, treatment and course of the illness. The belief about the cause and effective treatment options for mental illness is usually understood in a variety of ways by different cultures. While the number of people with mental illness has continued to increase worldwide, access to treatment has continued to decline.

In Nigeria, more than 90% of people with serious mental illness do not have access to medical treatment. This has been attributed to paucity of medical health care workers and lack of facilities especially in rural communities. While most medical treatment facilities are located in urban centres, majority of the people reside in rural communities. Consequently, it is estimated that more than 80% of people with mental illness seek care from alternative sources including traditional and spiritual healers. Other factors such as stigma, poverty, low literacy level, ignorance, and lack of belief in the efficacy of orthodox treatment have made traditional treatment an important component of mental health care in most communities.

HISTORY

Care of people with mental illness among the Yoruba ethnic group of South Western Nigeria predates the advent of orthodox medicine in Yorubaland. A major determinant of choice of treatment among sick people is belief about the cause of the illness. Where a sick person or his family do not agree with the therapist about the cause of illness, there is lack of trust in the efficacy of the treatment. In Yoruba culture, traditional healers are important component of mental health care because their belief system compliments the prevailing cultural beliefs of the people regarding causes of mental illness.

Traditional care of people with mental illness are based on the belief that psychiatric illnesses are caused by supernatural forces punishing the sick person or his family. Mental illness is frequently attributed to culturally acceptable beliefs about divinity, witchcraft, influence of ancestral spirit and social wrongdoing. Consequently, many people prefer traditional medicine as a primary source of mental health care. It is estimated that more than 80% of individuals and families seek mental health care from traditional healers, religious homes and spiritualists. However, where orthodox mental health services are available, people may migrate between orthodox and traditional mental health care.

Traditional healers may exist as individuals or group of healers organized with rules governing their association. In our environment, traditional healers outnumber orthodox medical practitioners. This can be attributed to the ease with which people attain the status of a traditional healer. There is little or no training, no designated duration for qualification and qualification acquired by inheritance. This form of care has continued to exist and develop concurrently with orthodox medical care among Yoruba people. In contrast, orthodox mental health care workers require many years of training to obtain qualification to practice. They have strict practice ethics and regulations by professional licensing bodies and associations. These make traditional mental health care services more available, accessible and cheaper than orthodox medicine.

DIAGNOSIS

Yoruba people have description for various mental illnesses which most times depict the symptoms of the illness. Local terminologies such as *Ode Ori* (heat, peppery or crawling sensation in the head), *Asiwin* (madness), *Aganna* (psychosis due to infection or medical illness such as severe malaria), *Abisiwin* (psychosis after childbirth), *Didirin* (mental retardation), *Were* (psychosis), and *Warapa* (eplipesy) have been used to describe mental disorders. These terminologies were not documented in written form but passed on verbally through successive generations of traditional healers.

In orthodox medicine, mental illnesses are classified into groups each with specific constellation of symptoms and signs as recommended by committee of mental health experts. These include schizophrenia, mania, bipolar disorder, depression, dementia and delirium among others. However, this classification is not recognized among Yoruba traditional healers.

Traditional healers determine the nature or diagnosis of mental illness through interviews, history taking, spiritual supplication, divination and prayers. In Yoruba traditional care for mental health problems, divination and consultation with the spirit world play important role. Many people believe treatment of mental illness is beyond the capacity of orthodox medicine.

On the other hand, orthodox medicine uses classification systems which set out criteria required to make a diagnosis of specific mental illness. These include the eleventh version of International Classification of Diseases (ICD 11) by the World Health Organization and the Diagnostic and Statistical Manual of the American Psychiatric Association.

TREATMENT

Evolution of traditional care for mental illnesses among Yoruba people was similar to the development of orthodox medicine. Early treatment involved rituals, offerings to appease the gods or for atonement for wrong doings, incisions to release evil spirit and herbal treatment. One of the commonly used herbs is the Rauwolfia plant used as tranquilizer to treat people with psychotic symptoms. Extract from roots, bark and leaves of this tropical plant (Rauwolfia vomituria) which is called "**Ewe Asofeyeje**" in Yoruba language is used in the treatment of mentally ill people. Traditional healers recognize that psychiatric illness can be caused by physical ailments such as severe malaria, substance abuse, head trauma and stress of difficult labour during childbirth among others. Similar to orthodox treatment, traditional care of the mentally ill include both pharmacological and non-pharmacological methods.

The former include use of herbs, incisions, and hydrotherapy while the latter consists of prayers, fasting, sacrifices, rituals, incantations, chants, counselling and psychotherapy among others. The waiting time is short because the number of clients is usually small compared to the number of practitioners and time spent for consultation is short. Cost of treatment is usually within the reach of the people in the community. Payment is made easy as clients are allowed to pay in affordable instalments.

Traditional healers often provide acceptable explanations about the nature and cause of the illness to their clients. They offer acceptable explanation about the individual symptoms, the cause of the illness and treatment options that aligns with the person's beliefs about mental illness. These community based healers have deep personal involvement in the healing process and explain illness in terms of social interaction and spirituality. This practice presents a holistic concept of mental illness and is more consistent with the culture of the people. Treatment takes place mostly within the community and it involves the family of the sick person. These attributes endeared many people to traditional treatment.

Orthodox mental health care is currently saddled with an array of challenges especially funding and availability of qualified professionals as the country struggles with mass exodus of medical professionals. Other challenges making orthodox treatment less desirable include long waiting time, unmotivated workforce, high cost of treatment and lack of cultural components in service delivery. The waiting time is long and some clients spend virtually the whole day accessing care especially in busy public hospitals. The staffs are poorly trained, poorly paid and unmotivated. The staffs sometimes are inconsiderate and disrespectful to clients because they believe they are rendering special assistance. Clients are frequently not informed about the nature of their illness and treatment options available. In most hospitals and clinics, cost of treatments is expensive and not affordable for most people.

The process of accessing treatment is cumbersome even in hospitals where treatment is highly subsidized. Treatment focuses basically on the physical symptoms of the client with little or no attention paid to spiritual aspect of the illness. In orthodox care, clients are separated from their culture, home, family, friends and community as they stay in hospital. Yoruba people prefer community-based treatment as opposed to hospital care which takes place away from home, family and friends in an unfamiliar environment.

Introduction of orthodox care for the mentally ill has eroded the roles of the family in the care of the sick. This has resulted in loss of benefits a familiar therapeutic environment confers on individuals on treatment for mental disorders. Professor Adeoye Lambo, recognizing the importance of communal life in management of mental illnesses, set up the 'Village System' in Aro, Abeokuta where mental health care was provided with family members staying in the facility along with sick person to ensure comprehensive care in a familiar environment. Similarly, traditional healers have introduced certain orthodox practices to their profession with the aim to modernize traditional medicine. These include consultation, investigations, diagnosis and treatment using a combination of orthodox methods and traditional practice.

There have been reports of human rights violation in traditional mental health care including physical restrains, isolation, starving, rituals, sacrificial offerings and exorcism. While human rights abuse in orthodox mental health care is uncommon and presently illegal following the recent signing of the Mental Health Bill 2022 into law, individuals with mental illness are vulnerable to violation of their Rights either in orthodox or traditional mental health care.

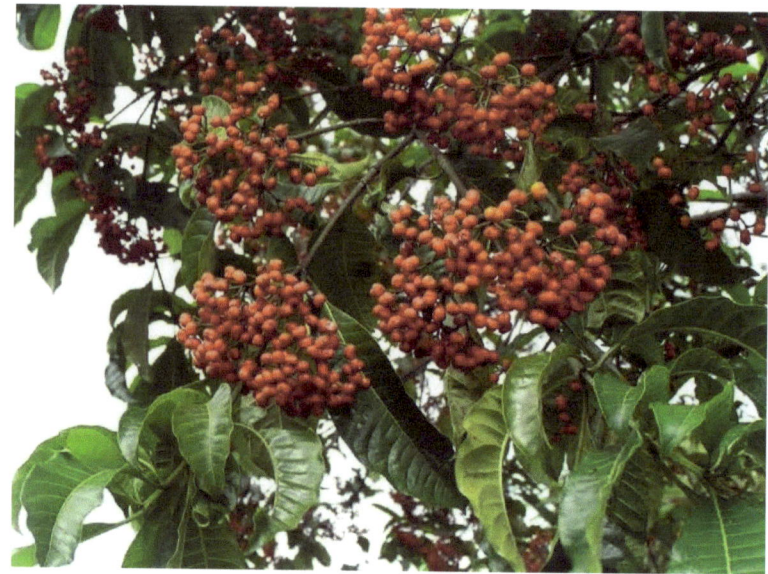

Poison devil's pepper (Rauwolfia vomituria) which is called "**Ewe Asofeyeje**" in Yoruba language is used in the traditional treatment of mentally ill people.

COLLABORATION

Although desirable, it has not been possible to develop collaboration between traditional and orthodox mental health care. This can be attributed to lack of understanding and faith in alternative treatment option. Traditional healers do not have faith in the efficacy of orthodox medical treatment because they regard the cause of mental illness as spiritual and not medical. Similarly, orthodox medical practitioners regard traditional medicine as archaic, obsolete, non-efficacious and even dangerous since it has no empirical basis.

Provision of acceptable, accessible, and affordable mental health services requires integration of traditional mental health care to the mental health care of the country. Orthodox treatment is grossly inadequate to provide required services for the large population especially in the rural areas where mental health workers and facilities are in short supply. It is essential that modern psychiatric knowledge and skills are integrated into existing traditional mental health care services.

Although considered crude and unsophisticated by many, traditional mental health care is an integral part of mental health service delivery among Yoruba ethnic group. It has major challenges of non-documentation of services for the purpose of provision of medical services, follow-up treatment or data for research. Improvement of documentation of history, procedures and treatment offered to people will make traditional mental health care more desirable.

In addition, traditional healers require mental education and training. Required areas of training include importance of collaboration with orthodox medicine, patient engagement, identification of symptoms of mental illness and treatment. Research on practice of traditional mental health care is also required to provide empirical basis for its therapeutic principles especially its safety and efficacy.

References

1. Raymond Prince (2006). The use of Rauwolfia for the treatment of psychoses by Nigerian Native doctors. The American Journal of Psychiatry.
2. Anjorin O and Wada, Y.H. (2022). Impact of traditional healers in the provision of mental health services in Nigeria. Annals of Medicine and Surgery. 82:104755.
3. Agara A.J., Makanjuola A.B., Morakinyo O. Management of perceived mental health problems by spiritual healers: A Nigerian study. Afr. J. psychiatry. 2008;11(2):113-118.
4. WHO (2010). MhGAP. Geneva: World Health Organization.

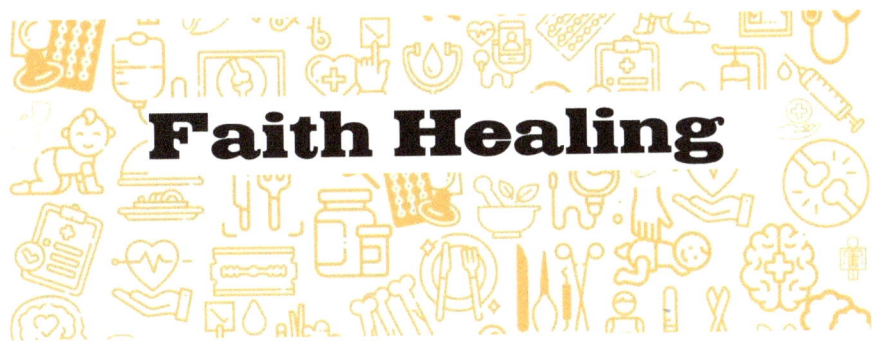

Faith Healing

10

Faith healing or **divine healing** is a term commonly used in Pentecostal churches. The term can be defined as healing of diseases through prayers and other acts like laying-on of hands. Some pastors are said to have the gift of faith healing because when they pray for people, healings are said to take place.

Outside the church, healing of diseases are said to occur in other spiritual settings. Such spiritual settings could be that of the traditional healer (called *Babalawo* among the *Yorubas*), Islamic clerics, and other practitioners of various religions. These sets of people may use incantations and spiritual materials on people to bring about healings.

Orthodox medicine is based upon science. Diseases are diagnosed based upon scientific practices. The diagnosis of a disease starts with the patient stating his complaints. Thereafter, the medical practitioner physically examines the patient. A few diseases can be diagnosed and treated at this stage. But special investigations like laboratory tests of body specimens, such as blood, stool, urine and radiological tests may be required to confirm the diagnosis. It is after a proper diagnosis is done that appropriate treatment is commenced. There is no secrecy in the various steps taken in the management of the disease and such steps can be repeated by other practitioners elsewhere. This is not the normal practice in *faith healing*. The whole process is centred on the healer alone and it is usually secretive. In the church, the outcome of treatment is at times ascribed to the sick person's faith. It is often said that the failure of the healing process is due to the faithlessness of the sick person.

The beauty of orthodox medicine is the openness and the recognition that not all diseases are curable. Advances in science enable improved methods of treatment of diseases from time to time.

My parents attended a Pentecostal church (The Apostolic Church) during their life-time; hence, I was exposed to faith healing through prayers early in life. I can remember an occasion in my primary school days when I encouraged my father to pray for a sibling of mine who had fever and rigors, instead of going to buy him **Cafenol**, the commonly - used analgesic. However, I stopped living with my parents during my secondary school days as I was in the boarding house throughout in Anglican schools. My belief in the idea of faith healing therefore became weakened. Probably, I would have been discouraged from studying medicine in the University if I had remained at home with my parents throughout. Can this be explained as destiny?

In my senior classes in the secondary school, I came in contact with Christians who belonged to The Apostolic Faith. One of the tenets of the church is **faith healing**. Members do not go to the hospital for medical treatment whenever they fall ill. Any sick person would be prayed for in the church and is expected to recover from ill-health. Over the years, I attended burial ceremonies of some of their members. I observed that many of them appeared joyful saying their brother/sister has gone to heaven.

As a Christian myself, claiming heaven was not strange to me, but this manner was not clear to me. A usual bible quotation at such burial ceremonies was 2nd Timothy 4:7-8 where Apostle Paul stated that he had fought a good fight and that a crown of righteousness awaited him on the day of judgment. Later, I learnt that converted medical workers (doctors and nurses) have to confess the 'sin of medical practice' and go to other professional fields. This appeared totally disagreeable to me as a medical practitioner.

I got closer to the members of the church in the 1990s when I rented a house built by one of its members. I then observed that herbal concoctions could be taken by sick members but that they must not take orthodox medicines. Over the years, I have noticed many of their members coming to the hospital for medical treatment albeit without the official permission of the church.

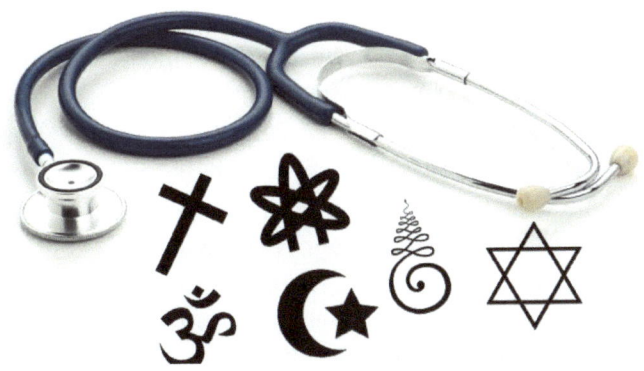

Faith healing versus orthodox medicine.

During my days in the secondary school and the university, I attended the Anglican Church which does not practice **divine healing**. A few years into my marriage in 1985, my father visited me and convinced me to start attending The Apostolic Church. Earlier, a close relative, Uncle Sam Ojo, invited me to be attending the Apostolic Church but I was reluctant. I was surprised when he later asked me to treat a senior pastor in his local parish. The pastor gladly accepted injections and tablets from me, contrary to my earlier perception of The Apostolic Church where they would rather pray for a sick person instead of taking him to the hospital for orthodox medical treatment. I thereafter followed the advice of my father and started attending the Apostolic Church with my family. I was well received by the church and have been of help to many members and pastors. I even heard a former head of the Church expressing that there was nothing wrong with orthodox medicine but that leaders of the church chose **divine healing** during the colonial days so as to discourage members from going back to pagan worship and sacrifices in the process of seeking for healing outside the church.

Before the death of my father, he told me stories of many sick members who died because they refused to go to the hospital for orthodox medical treatment. Some of these people were accused by pastors of falling ill because they had failed in the payment of tithes to the Church and that the relatives would be compelled to pay the amount owed. I would then ask him if such people got healed but his response was that they never recovered.

In present day Nigeria, I believe it is only The Apostolic Faith Church that still preaches divine healing alone as all others believe in orthodox medicine. Many churches have even gone ahead to build hospitals where orthodox medicine is being practiced. In the Redeemed Christian Church of God where I now worship, we run clinics for the medically sick. I join fellow medical practitioners at the Medical Centre of the Redemption Camp whenever I go there for the monthly Holy Ghost Services. Medical Outreaches are done by the Church as a welfare outreach to communities and at the regular Let's-Go-A-Fishing (evangelistic) programs.

In addition, I shall briefly discuss the Jehovah's Witness, which is a distinct sect in Christianity. They have branches in many countries and are known to have clashes with government regulations. I grew up to know of the sect as a child as they always go about preaching and distributing religious books. One of their major tenets is their refusal to accept blood transfusion when they come for medical treatment in hospitals. There is usually loss of blood in surgeries and this is of importance to surgeons. **Having practiced surgery within and outside Nigeria, I have observed that Africans (Negroids) tend to bleed more than Caucasians and Asians during surgery**. Many of my colleagues who have practiced in Africa and Europe have made a similar observation.

After blood loss from surgery or any other cause, the human body may be able to cope and replace such losses up to a certain level. However, a significant blood loss at a time may compromise the haemodynamics of the cardiovascular system if the loss is much. Thus, the heart may not be able to pump blood adequately to all organs and tissues of the body. Failure of organs may result which can ultimately result in the death of the individual. A surgeon will not be happy if death results after an otherwise successful surgery. Jehovah's Witnesses most often have disagreements with orthodox medical practitioners when there is need for blood transfusion. Many medical practitioners will simply refuse to treat Jehovah's Witnesses who may need blood transfusion in the course of the treatment.

For me as a surgeon, I try to be understanding when Jehovah's Witnesses present for medical treatment. Conservation of blood and limiting blood loss are part of the fundamental training of a surgeon. Blood transfusion is risky and I have witnessed some patients dying from blood reaction. We practitioners tend to recommend blood transfusion as a desperate attempt to save the life of the patient. Blood substitutes are available but most of them cannot replace the natural functions of the blood inside the human body. Whenever I am performing surgery on a patient who refuses blood transfusion, I am extra careful in controlling bleeding. It gladdens my heart to say that I have had successes in most cases. I would not blame any medical practitioner who refuses to treat Jehovah's Witnesses who may require blood transfusion during treatment.

Since I treat members of the Jehovah's Witness sect from time to time, I have been exposed to literature materials on the doctrine of the sect and scientific papers on blood substitutes and processes of boosting blood in the human body. However, the Biblical basis for refusal of blood transfusion intrigues me as a Christian. The scriptural basis for Jehovah's Witnesses refusal of blood transfusion is from the Acts of the Apostles 15: 29 – *"That ye abstain from meats offered to idols, **and from blood**, and from things strangled, and from fornication; from which if ye keep yourselves, ye shall do well. Fare ye well."*

From Church history, we learnt that there was a Jerusalem Council Meeting by the Apostles following the spread of the gospel to the gentiles. Despite the fact that the gentiles were accepting Christ and receiving the Baptism of the Holy Spirit, some Apostles and early missionaries believed and taught that the gentile Christians must be converted to Judaism (circumcised) before they could be accepted. But the Council meeting only gave the recommendation quoted above. God's instructions to the Jews concerning sacrifices and blood can be found in Leviticus 17: 10-16. Dakes' Annotated Reference Bible explains "abstain from blood" thus – 'This not only includes eating blood, but all cruelty and murder in its various forms.' May be the practice then was to strangulate the animal and cook with the blood to sweeten it. But God frowned against this.

In our clime, it is the normal practice to slaughter the animal and let out the blood. Thus 'eating of blood' is not a common practice. Even animals killed by hunters in the bush have the blood washed out from the meat before cooking for consumption.

Extension of the issue of 'abstaining from blood' to medical treatment appears rather far-fetched to my Christian mind. As of the period the scriptures were written more than 2,000 years ago, orthodox medical treatment had not developed. The use of blood transfusion for medical treatment only developed during the early part of the 20th century (i.e. about 100 years ago). I believe strongly that the instruction on abstaining from blood refers to animal sacrifices rather than medical treatment.

All physicians, and particularly surgeons, know that every attempt should be made to conserve the patient's blood and many methods have been developed on how to do this. Transfusion of blood may create problems such as blood reactions and transmission of infections. Efforts are made to properly screen the blood and cross-match in the laboratory before the blood is transfused. The medical adage is that the best blood is the patient's blood. It is obvious therefore that the use of blood for transfusion in medical practice is a desperate attempt to save life.

I accept to treat Jehovah's Witnesses and have taken the risk many times. Those of them who refuse blood transfusion are humans and must be cared for. Luckily enough, most of the cases I have handled have survived, even if they have to stay longer on admission than necessary in building up their blood levels.

As a Christian and an orthodox medical practitioner, I believe in the scientific basis of diseases and do practice accordingly. However, I do pray for success at my professional practice and also pray for recovery of my patients. I also believe that certain illnesses may have spiritual input; either the right help will not come or unexpected complications may arise and these may not be easily explained. But I struggle to investigate scientifically all illnesses before considering spiritual inputs or causes. Thus, I believe that praying for patients is quite helpful, even in orthodox medical practice.

In summary, it is obvious that orthodox medical practice is superior to African traditional medical practice in the management of most diseases. I, therefore, encourage the general populace to seek appropriate help when faced with medical conditions.

References.

1. Village, Andrew (2005). "Dimensions of belief about miraculous healing". Mental Health, Religion & Culture. 8 (2): 97-107.

2. Kalb, Claudia (2003-11-09). "Faith & Healing. Newsweek. 142(19): 44-50, 53-54, 56.

3. Asser, Seth M.; Swan Rita (April 1998). "Child fatalities from religion-motivated medical nelect". Pediatrics. 101 (4):625-629.

4. The Holy Bible. King James Version.

5. Dakes Annotated Reference Bible. By Finnis Jennings Dake. Dake Publishing, Inc. 2001.

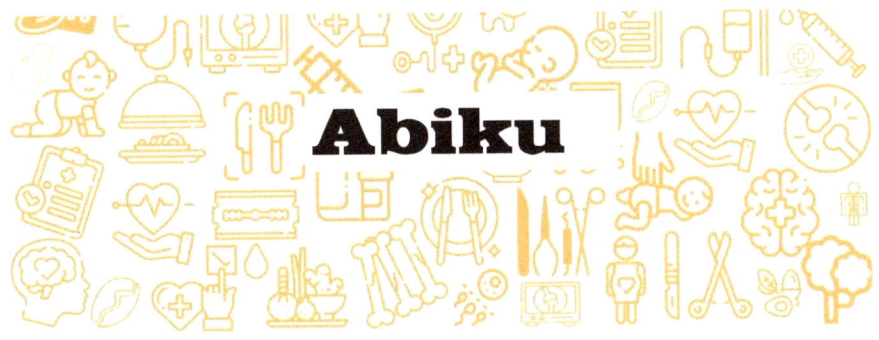

Abiku

11

***ABIKU* – My Personal Experience.**

Abiku is a myth in Yoruba land that persisted for centuries but faded out with the advent of Western Orthodox Medicine. As the name implies, it means a child that dies soon after delivery or a child that dies before reaching puberty. The child soon comes back to the world and most often is re-born by the same mother. The process of death and re-birth is repeated over and over. It is regarded as a spiritual affliction of women. For example, a woman could have had several deliveries yet only a few will grow into adulthood. In previous centuries, some women were so unlucky that all the children they gave birth to would die in infancy.

At a personal level, my mother must have given birth to 7 or 8 children, but only 3 of us survived into adulthood – myself, born in 1952, Lydia, born in 1959 and Oluyinka, born in 1963. The first incident I remember is my mother giving birth to a male child before Lydia was born: the boy was some months old when he died and my father's aunt, Mama Alice, was called to bury the baby. The baby was flogged with a broomstick before burial and I saw the boy urinating during the process. I believe the whipping was to ward off the spirit of *Abiku* so that he would not come back again and repeat the circle of being born and dying in infancy. Marks may be made on the faces and bodies of children who are regarded as Abikus. We had tales of children being born with some of the marks they were given in early lives. However, I was too young to confirm some of these stories.

Another incident occurred after Oluyinka was born. I remember my mother having premature delivery of twins that never survived. I was not told the details but I believe that my mother died in 1969 trying to have more children. It was not surprising that my father married a second wife soon after Lydia was born. The pressure on him must have been much as the first wife could only give him two (2) children after ten (10) years of marriage. The decision must have been tough for him because he was a member of The Apostolic Church which frowns on polygamy. A polygamous man is not regarded as a church member, and if a member, he would be suspended which meant he could not partake in the Holy Communion or be ordained as a Deacon or Elder. I remember my mother taking part in the sharing of the Holy Communion in the church as the first wife. The second wife was not qualified to be a member of the church. My father remained a member of the Apostolic Church throughout his lifetime.

Many marriages must have been affected by the *Abiku* condition. Polygamy was common back then as a means to have many children as in my father's case. A hallmark of a successful man in Yoruba land was having many children. The importance of this was that having many children meant having more hands to work on the farm, whether in planting, weeding or harvesting.

A generation after, the believe in *Abiku* has disappeared as most children born survive into adulthood. The reasons are obvious – vaccination, education and improved standard of living and increased availability of modern medical services generally.

a. **Vaccination**

   Vaccinations against most childhood diseases have been available at various local government health centres since the early 1970s and were often free. The vaccines are BCG against Tuberculosis, Diphtheria, Pertussis, Tetanus, and Measles during infancy, etc. There are also vaccines available for adults, like those for Tetanus and Rabies.

b. **Education and improved standard of living**

In the 1950s and 1960s, few individuals in Nigeria had any formal education; few had secondary school education, and fewer had tertiary education. However, the level of education in the country has improved considerably in recent decades. Better education means increased knowledge which includes health education. In addition, many taboos have been broken or discarded as a result of Western education. Good education translates into good earning powers for families and improved living. High-quality foods are more expensive than cheaper starchy foods which can easily be purchased for the home. There is also improved knowledge of the quality of food that the growing bodies of children require. In those days, our parents depended more on tradition and myths passed from generation to generation.

An example I remember from my childhood is that children were forbidden from eating chicken eggs. We were told that children who ate eggs would become thieves. I am sure no educated parents would forbid their children from eating chicken eggs. Scientifically, a chicken egg is a complete meal loaded with protein that growing children need.

I also observed then that only the male heads of family units ate meat. The children would be lucky to have meat left over by the elders to eat or have their mother share tiny pieces among the then. Parents did not know that it is the children who require large amounts of protein for their growing bodies. The kinds of foods we ate in our growing up years were mainly starchy with little or no protein necessary for good body growth.

c. **Inadequacy or Non-availability of Hospitals and Health Care Centres**

There were very few hospitals in my growing up years in the 1950s and 1960s. As a result, most ailments were treated at home, based on whatever local facilities were available or the traditional medical practices. My father once told me the story of how he lost a male toddler. This must have been in the years before my sister, Lydia, was born. He described the boy as chubby and beautiful. The boy only had a skin rash and my father was advised to take him for treatment at a patent medicine shop known as *Gaskiya*. The boy was given an injection and died instantly, possibly due to a drug reaction or wrong administration.

I knew *Gaskiya* Patent Medicine shop very well. It was located in the centre of the town close to the Police Station. I must have been sent there a few times to buy some tablets. The only tablet I can remember buying was a sulphonamide used in treating wounds. The name was barely mentioned and was nicknamed *'Monu'* (secret). *Gaskiya* was not a skilled health worker.

The care of wounds during my growing-up years was poor. Most of us primary school children went to school bare-footed. A few parents bought shoes for their children to be worn during the festivals or to attend church services on Sundays. Walking bare-footed made the individual susceptible to injuries, particularly on the toes. I have a few deformed toes and scars from the numerous wounds I had in my early years.

As primary school children, we treated fresh wounds with saliva applied to paper or plant leaves. If the wounds became big, our parents would notice and then sent us for wound dressings at the home of a nurse or dispensary assistant. In my home town, *Baba Alamu* was quite popular and had no rival in the care of wounds. We would go to his house early in the morning on our way to school for wound dressings. I can remember *Baba Alamu* using pinkish-looking water to clean the wounds by applying cotton wool on which he would apply a cream and a white powder. I believe the pinkish water had potassium permanganate and the powder must have been penicillin powder. The wounds took time to heal and we did not have tetanus vaccines then.

I remember sustaining two big wounds in the early 1960s and my father had to apply different treatments. The first wound was a deep nail puncture wound I sustained in the children's church that was under construction. I could not walk about for a while and my father was applying undiluted *Izal* disinfectant to the deep wound. The wound later healed.

The second wound was sustained on the farm in 1965 when Rashidi, my father's tailoring apprentice, and I were pursuing a rat. I got to the rat first and while I was trying to hit it, the cutlass was caught up by a creeper on the cocoa farm. Since the rat was right in front of me, I attempted to grab the rat with my bare hands. Unfortunately, my partner brought his cutlass down on my two wrists. I sustained big wounds on both wrists that bled heavily. To stop the bleeding, we applied juice from cut plantain suckers. The bleeding soon stopped but I still had big wounds on my wrists. I was afraid of being beaten by my father and so I hid till night before returning to our family hut in the village. By this time, the wounds had become so painful. For treatment, my father used a cream made with the sap of *'Arere'* tree mixed with red palm oil. The wounds healed after a while. I still have the transverse scars on the back of each wrist as a reminder. I also have a number of scars on the shin of both legs as a reminder of the various wounds I sustained in my early years.

The common vaccination available then was Small Pox Vaccination. The World Health Organization organized mass vaccination globally. For the children, the health team would visit primary schools. The school gate would be shut to prevent pupils from running away for fear of taking injections. We lined up on the playing field to be vaccinated. The vaccine was applied to the upper left arm. There were two modes of administration:

- Long sharp needles were used to scratch the skin and the vaccine was applied as a topical cream.
- Gun-like nozzles delivered the vaccine into punched holes in the skin.

Both methods of vaccine delivery were painful. I must have received the vaccination up to 2 or 3 times leaving a scar on my left arm. The mass Immunization against Small Pox was successful with the eradication of Small Pox worldwide in 1977.

'Ṣọ̀pọ̀na', as smallpox was called, was worshipped as a deity by the Yoruba people. The name was only said in a hushed tone or it was simply called 'Baba'. Some adherents worshipped the deity. During outbreaks of smallpox, the adherents were usually busy. They would bury whoever died from smallpox and inherit the property of the deceased. Later in the Medical School, I learnt that adherents of Ṣọ̀pọ̀na immunized themselves by getting exposed to low doses of the dust collected from the dwellings of sufferers. These adherents are said to have started epidemics by spreading this special dust around the neighbourhoods.

There was an epidemic of smallpox in our village, *Ogundijo*, about the mid-1960s. Families had to abandon their farms and relocate to the town. I remember my father discussing this with Pa Olanrewaju, our next-door neighbour in the town. He told his neighbour that they had been spraying **Izal** disinfectant inside the houses and surroundings. Isolation and social distancing which were used to limit the spread of the most recent pandemic, Covid-19, were also in our cultural practice.

Our people recognized the medicinal value of honey. I remember my father applying honey to my head to treat a fungal infection, *Tinea capitis*, in the early 1960s. House flies were following me about but I enjoyed scrapping the honey with my fingers and licking it. Of course, the fungal infection cleared.

Many years later, I learnt about the efficacy of honey in the treatment of wounds from publications of my erstwhile flat mate at the Wesley Guild Hospital, Ilesha, during my Internship, Professor Fashika of the University College Hospital, Ibadan, in the 1990s. Consequently, as an experienced surgeon, I use honey a lot in the treatment of wounds.

d. Many children must have been born with sickle cell disease and not many would survive till adulthood with the dearth of health centres. The average child with sickle cell disease goes into crisis easily and the best treatment they would have was concoctions. For an already compromised liver, liver failure and death would be the end result most times.

In modern times, the average educated family is aware of the fact that marriage between couples whose genotype is AS results in birthing children with sickle cell disease. Many churches in Nigeria counsel young people on the need to check their genotypes before marriage and some even refuse to join affected couples in holy matrimony. Thus the number of children with sickle cell disease is reducing generally in the general population. And with the availability of good health centres the care of children born with sickle cell disease has improved and many of such children now survive into adulthood.

References.

1. Timothy Mobolade. "The Concept of Abiku" African Arts. Vol. 7.No. 1 (1973), pp. 62-64.
2. John Pepper Clark. (1965) Abiku (Spirit Child).

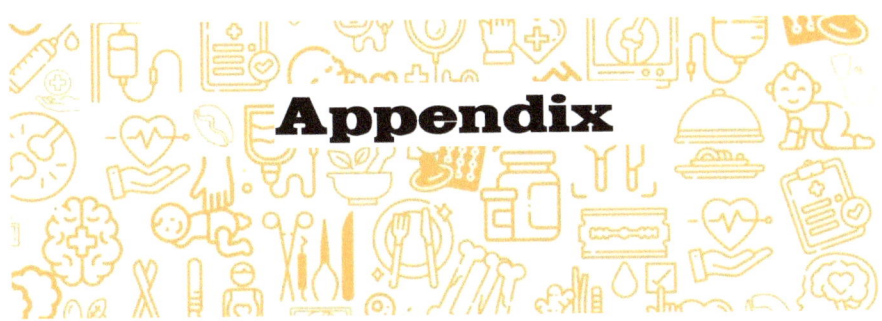

Appendix

(In memory of my late father, Pa James Bolarinwa Odetayo who had facial marks, I have decided to add this write-up on Tribal Marks.)

TRIBAL MARKS IN YORUBALAND
BY PETER TAIWO ODETAYO B.A. (Hons)

The history of tribal marks among the Yorubas cannot be traced to a particular period. According to the great Yoruba historian, Professor Adeboye Babalola in his book, *Ása ati Ise Ile Yoruba*, the practice is as old as the word *Yoruba*. An agreement on who started it has not been reached among scholars. Tribal marks are scarifications designed to beautify and identify a particular set of people. It is a laceration made on the face or body and can be vertically, horizontally and diagonally designed, depending on the family and community who instituted it.

Tribal marks are made through a scarification technique by the beautician called *Oloola*. This beautician usually uses metals or sharp objects, such as razor blades, to inscribe the marks and concoctions for pain relief and quick healing of the wounds. It is important to note that in Yorubaland, the *Oloola* is a professional.

THE HISTORY OF TRIBAL MARKS IN YORUBALAND

The first oral tradition is that King *Sango* of the old Oyo Empire initiated tribal marks. The death of his mother at a tender age prevented him from knowing her and associating with her. He had to perform a sacrifice for the spirit of his late mother but, unfortunately, he did not know her name. He sent two servants to his matrilineal home in *Tapa* Land to inquire about the name of his mother and offer sacrifice. The servants were well received with food and drinks, but in the process, one of the servants got drunk and could not participate in the sacrifice.

Upon their return home, King Sango was very bitter about the drunk servant and punished him by inscribing marks on his face as a reward for his disgraceful act. However, the marks on his face beautified him the more. King Sango then commanded all his princes and princesses to pass through the same process.

On seeing this as well, the Oyo high chiefs known as *Oyo Mesi*, equally subjected their children to the same process, but not the same marks, as a form of respect for the royal family. As a result of this development, it was decreed that all citizens of the Old – Oyo Empire must have marks depending on the agreed pattern.

The second oral tradition had it that the **Ifa** (the Yoruba god of divination) commanded the progenitor of the Yoruba race, *Oduduwa*, to inscribe tribal marks on all his children and followers before leaving Mecca for easy identification wherever they migrated. *Oduduwa* carried out the instruction and migrated to Ile-Ife while some of his children and followers migrated to different parts of the world. (It is noteworthy that certain tribes in Sudan, Egypt, Ethiopia and some parts of Northern Nigeria also have tribal marks similar to those of the Yorubas.)

This oral tradition helps us to understand that black people with tribal marks all over the world must have migrated with *Oduduwa* because they shared Yoruba culture and tradition. This means that they must have had a direct or indirect link with *Oduduwa*, the progenitor of the Yoruba race.

However, tribal marks have come to stay in *Yorubaland*, especially in *Oyo* town where the practice is still common despite increasing civilization. Even in the 21st century, any Oyo prince who wants to ascend the throne of his forefathers must be identified and beautified with tribal marks designed for the royal families.

TYPES OF TRIBAL MARKS IN YORUBALAND

There are six major tribal marks namely:

1. Abaja
2. Ture
3. Gombo
4. Yagba
5. Ila alagbara
6. Keke.

1. **Abaja**
   a. Abajakansoso
      Abajakansoso is a single vertical mark on each cheek. It is common among the Ondo people and its environs.

   b. Abaja meta ibule
      This consists of three horizontal marks on each cheek, starting from the ear to the mouth and usually located in the centre of the cheek. This tribal mark is common among the people of old Ile-Ife and the Igbomina.

   c. Abaja meta ooro (Pele)
      This is another distinctive tribal mark known as *Pele* among the Yorubas. It consists of three vertical marks on each cheek. *Abaja meta ooro* is commonly found among the Egba, Ife, Ijesa, Ila, Ibadan, Ijebu and Iseyin people.

2. This is another variant of *Abaja* with four horizontal marks on each cheek and it is commonly found among members of the families of the Bashorun chieftaincy title holders in Oyo town.

   a. Abaja merin ibule

   b. Abaja merin with baramu
      This variant of Abaja has four horizontal marks with a diagonal mark on each cheek. It is particular to the Oyo people.

c. Abaja mefa ibule/Abaja omo-oba Alaafin
This tribal mark is designed for the royal family in Oyo town. It consists of six horizontal marks broken into two equal groups with a small gap on each cheek.

d. Abaja meje
This consists of four horizontal marks and three vertical marks on each cheek. It is commonly found among the Oyo people.

e. Abaja mokanla
This variant of *Abaja* is also common among the people of Oyo town and it consists of eight horizontal marks divided into two groups and three vertical ones on each cheek.

f. Abaja Olowu
It consists of three vertical marks over three horizontal ones, which is common among the Olowu and Olofa families.

g. Abaja Ekiti
This variant of Abaja consists of twelve marks on a cheek, divided into nine horizontal marks and three vertical marks, out of which the nine horizontal ones are divided into three and the three vertical marks are placed over the horizontal ones.

3. Keke Olowu

This is a major tribal mark among the Owu people. It consists of small, but very bold, marks like incisions all over the face, starting from the ear down to the chin and coupled with three vertical marks on each face.

4. Ture

Ture tribal mark is popular in Yorubaland and the Northern part of Nigeria, especially in Borno among the Beriberi, Gogobiri and Daura people. This mark consists of four vertical marks beside the ear on each cheek with another three vertical marks very close to the nose but not as long as the initial four vertical ones.

5. Gombo

This is another stylish and prominent tribal mark in Yorubaland. *Gombo* is the combination of four horizontal and four vertical marks on each cheek with a gap between the two types.

6. **Gombo with baramu**

   This variant of *Gombo* is slightly different from real *Gombo* because there are four vertical and four horizontal marks coupled with a diagonal mark on each side of the face. This is common among the people of Ogbomoso in Oyo state.

7. **Abaja Efon**

   Abaja Efon is another variant of the *Abaja* group found among the Efon people of Osun and Ekiti states of South West Nigeria. *Abaja Efon* is characterized by small horizontal bold marks on both cheeks. One cannot easily identify the marks until the person moves closer.

8. **Ila alagbara (The Tribal Marks for the Wealthy)**

   If a princess marries from another clan or kingdom, the children born into such families will combine the tribal marks and their patrilineal and matrilineal homes as a form of respect for both families. Such tribal marks will be separated. The paternal tribal mark will be on the right cheek while the maternal tribal mark will be on the left cheek. This tribal mark is common among the ruling class and the wealthy among the Oyo people.

9. **Yagba**

   This mark consists of three diagonal marks right from the cheeks down to the mouth and it is common among the Yagba people who migrated from Ile-Ife.

Nowadays, the practice of giving children tribal marks is on the verge of extinction due to the influence of Western civilization brought by education and religion, particularly Christianity. Some governments even consider the practice as child abuse which is legislated against. Despite this, some communities still preserve this heritage and place much value on it, especially among the Oyos.

Dr. Olayioye Oluwole Odetayo

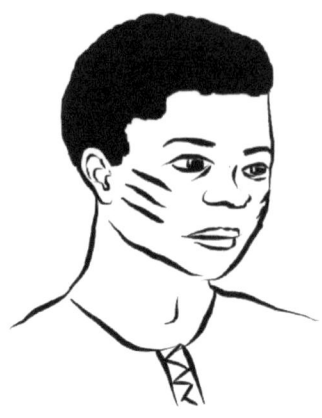 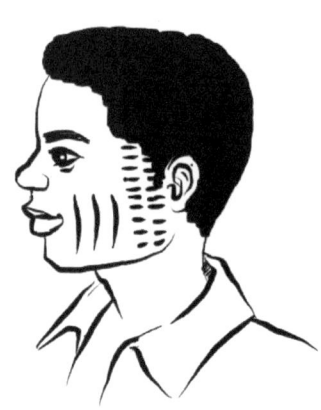

L- Àbajà mẹta Ibulẹ,
R- Kẹkẹ

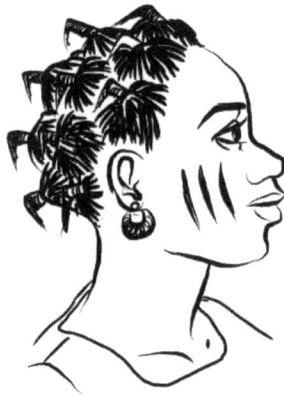 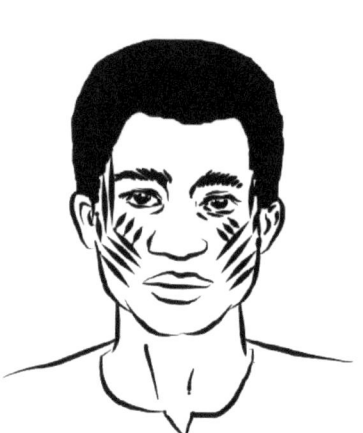

L- Pélé,
R- Gònbó àtí bààmí

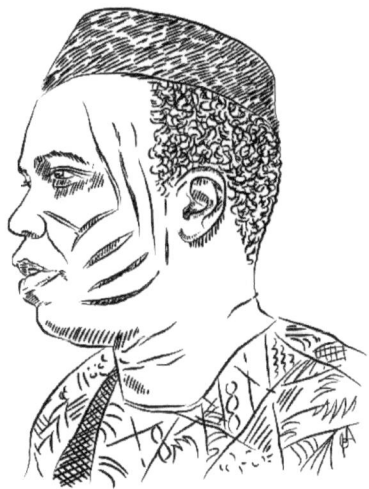

Yoruba man with tribal marks

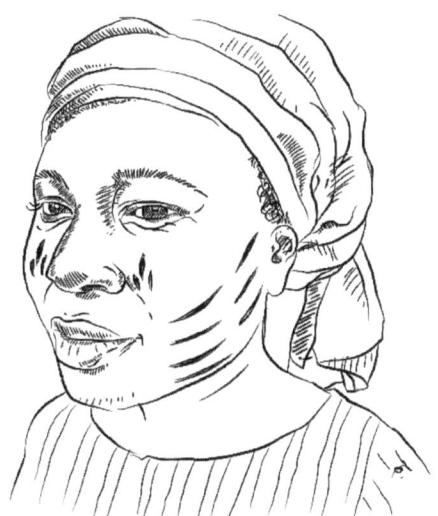

Yoruba woman with tribal marks

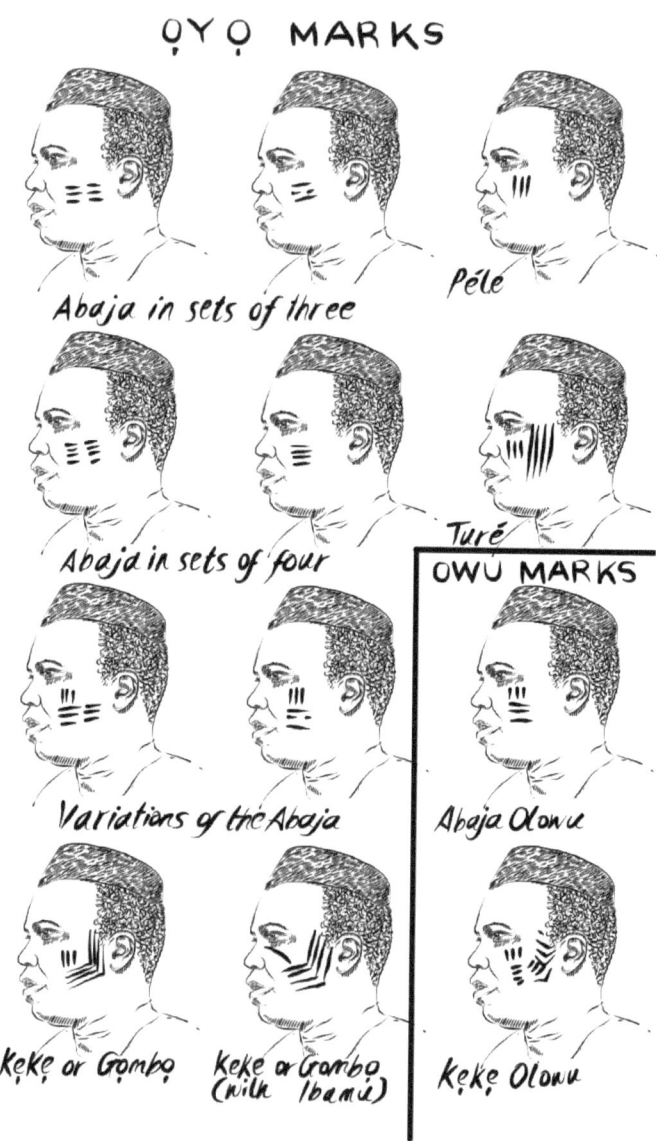

Tribal marks in Yorubaland

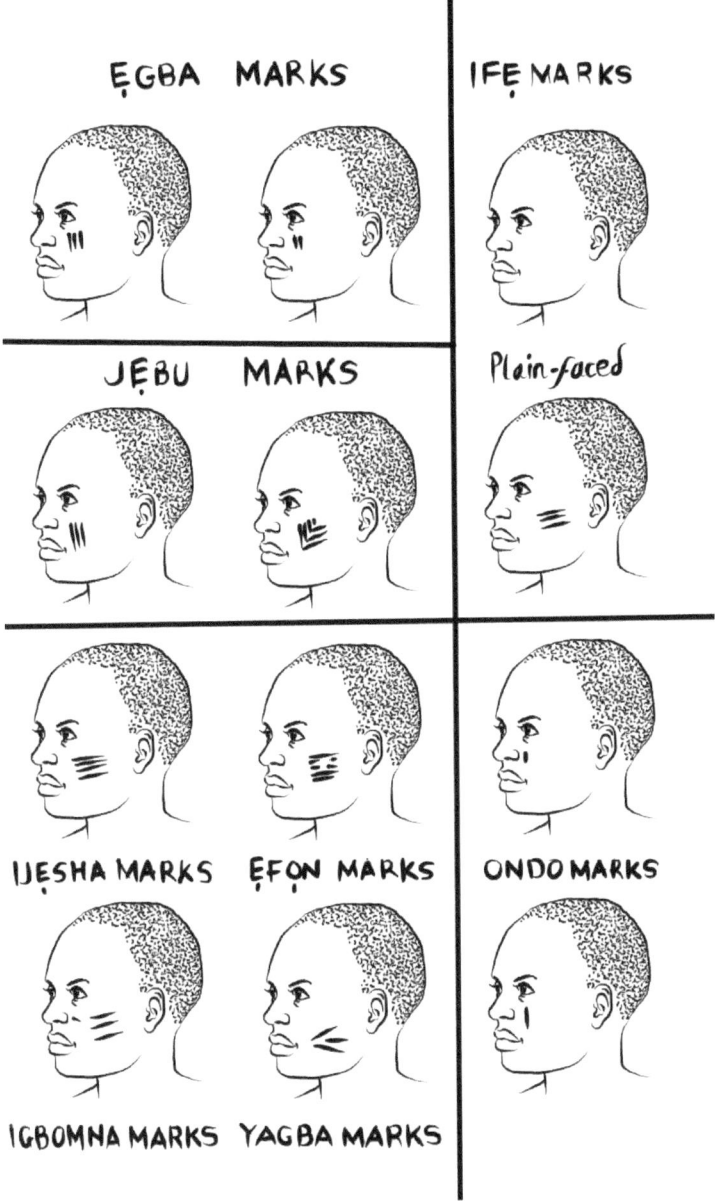

Tribal marks in Yorubaland

Dr. Olayioye Oluwole Odetayo

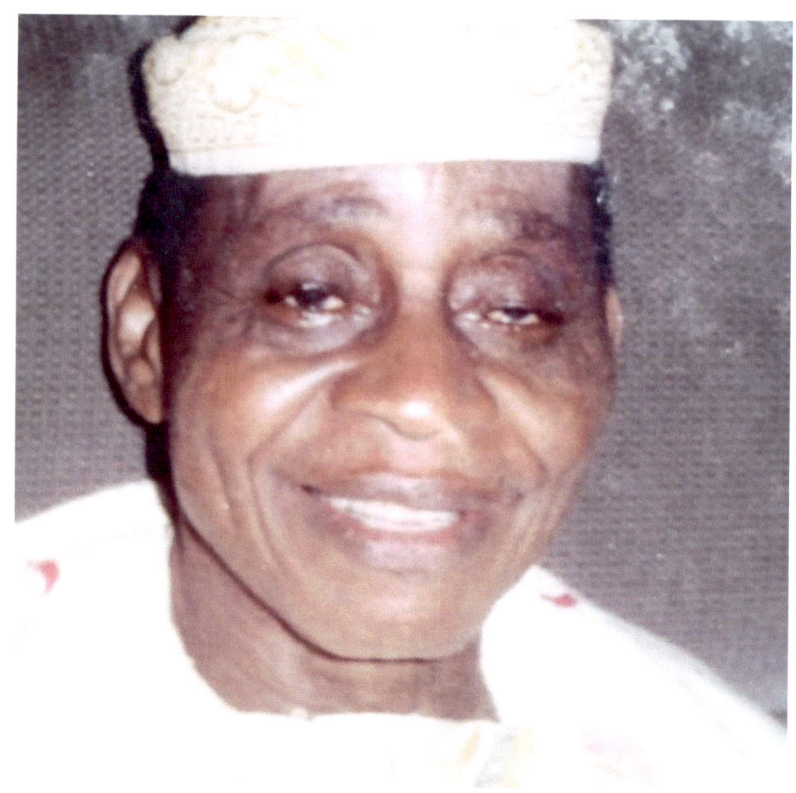

Late Pa James Bolarinwa Odetayo

References.

1. Usman, A. & Falola T. (2019) The Nineteeth Century Wars and Transformations. In the Yoruba from Prehistory to the Present (pp. 159-240). Cambridge: Cambridge University Press.
2. Bello, Abiodun. "Tribal marks, a people's identity. New Telegraph.
3. Mayaki, Victoria Ozohu. (2015). Nigeria: Tribal Marks – Our Lost Heritage" – All Africa.

Dr. Olayioye Oluwole Odetayo

ABOUT THE AUTHOR

Dr. Odetayo is a physician practicing in Lagos, Nigeria. He was born and nurtured by parents who are of ethnic Yoruba in the South-West, with strong cultural values. He attended primary and secondary schools run by the Anglican Mission before attending the University of Ife, now Obafemi Awolowo University, for his medical studies. He did the compulsory one year Internship before serving in the National Youth Service. Thereafter, he had his Residency (Postgraduate Studies) with the National Postgraduate Medical College of Nigeria. He successfully passed the final Fellowship Examinations in Surgery of the College in 1991.

He has held Consultant posts in Surgery in private and government hospitals in Nigeria. In the year 2000, he took up a Consultant Post in the Kingdom of Saudi Arabia for economic reasons. It is a common practice in many countries in Africa, for top professionals to emigrate to outside countries for improved remuneration. Since his return home in 2002, he runs his private hospital.

Dr. Odetayo is a family man with 4 grown-up children who are doing well in their chosen careers.

Dr. Olayioye Oluwole Odetayo

www.ingramcontent.com/pod-product-compliance
Lightning Source LLC
Chambersburg PA
CBHW041941240526
45473CB00033B/112